CLINICAL SKILLS FOR NURSING ADULTS

Sara Miller McCune founded SAGE Publishing in 1965 to suppo the dissemination of usable knowledge and educate a globa community. SAGE publishes more than 1000 journals and ove 800 new books each year, spanning a wide range of subject area Our growing selection of library products includes archives, dat case studies and video. SAGE remains majority owned by ou founder and after her lifetime will become owned by a charitab trust that secures the company's continued independence

Los Angeles | London | New Delhi | Singapore | Washington DC | Melbourr

CLINICAL SKILLS FOR NURSING ADULTS

STEP-BY-STEP

EDITED BY
WENDY WRIGHT, FIONA EVERETT AND PAUL NEWCOMBE

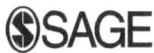

Los Angeles | London | New Delhi
Singapore | Washington DC | Melbourne

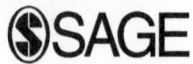

Los Angeles | London | New Delhi
Singapore | Washington DC | Melbourne

SAGE Publications Ltd
1 Oliver's Yard
55 City Road
London EC1Y 1SP

SAGE Publications Inc.
2455 Teller Road
Thousand Oaks, California 91320

SAGE Publications India Pvt Ltd
B 1/I 1 Mohan Cooperative Industrial Area
Mathura Road
New Delhi 110 044

SAGE Publications Asia–Pacific Pte Ltd
3 Church Street
#10-04 Samsung Hub
Singapore 049483

Editor: Alex Clabburn
Assistant editor: Jade Grogan
Production editor: Tanya Szwarnowska
Copyeditor: David Hemsley
Marketing manager: George Kimble
Cover design: Wendy Scott
Typeset by: C&M Digitals (P) Ltd, Chennai, India
Printed in the UK by Ashford Colour Press Ltd.

Library of Congress Control Number: 2018964614

British Library Cataloguing in Publication data

A catalogue record for this book is available from
the British Library

ISBN 978-1-4739-7577-4 (pbk)

At SAGE we take sustainability seriously. Most of our products are printed in the UK using responsibly sourced
papers and boards. When we print overseas we ensure sustainable papers are used as measured by the
PREPS grading system. We undertake an annual audit to monitor our sustainability.

CONTENTS

COMMON ABBREVIATIONS
WENDY WRIGHT AND FIONA EVERETT

Please note you may see the following abbreviations in practice. However, it is best practice to always use the full correct term to prevent mistakes and misunderstandings and to ensure patient safety.

ABG	Arterial blood gas
AF	Atrial fibrillation
BP	Blood pressure
C&S/ MC&S	Culture and sensitivity
CCU	Cardiac care unit / Coronary care unit
CO_2	Carbon dioxide
CPR	Cardiopulmonary resuscitation
CSU	Catheter specimen
CXR	Chest X-ray
DOB	Date of birth
DVT	Deep vein thrombosis
ECG	Electrocardiogram
EUA	Examination under anaesthetic
FBC	Full blood count
FBS	Fasting blood sugar
GCS	Glasgow Coma Scale
GI	Gastrointestinal
IM	Intramuscular
INR	International Normalized Ratio
IV	Intravenous
KVO	Keep vein open
MI	Myocardial infarction
MRI	Magnetic resonance imaging
MRSA	Meticillin-resistant Staphylococcus aureus

MSSU/MSU	Midstream specimen of urine
NAD	No abnormalities detected
NIDDM	Non insulin-dependent diabetes mellitus
NKA	No known allergies
NOK	Next of kin
NSAID	Non-steroidal anti-inflammatory drug
O_2	Oxygen
OT	Occupational therapist
PR	Per rectum
PRN	Pro re nata (when required)
PUO	Pyrexia of unknown origin
PV	Per vagina
SC	Subcutaneous
SOB	Shortness of breath
SpO_2	Peripheral capillary oxygen saturation
TIA	Transient ischaemic attack
TPR	Temperature, pulse, respiration
VS	Vital signs

USEFUL PREFIXES AND SUFFIXES

WENDY WRIGHT AND FIONA EVERETT

A e.g. asystole	Not, without, less
Ab, Abs e.g. abduction	From, away from
Ad e.g. adduction	Toward, in the direction of
Ambi e.g. ambidextrous	On both sides
Angi(o) e.g. angioplasty	Vessel
Ante e.g. antecedent	Before
Anti e.g. antibody	Against, opposing
Arteri(o) e.g. arteriosclerosis	Artery
Arthr(o) e.g. arthroplasty	Joint, articulation
Bi e.g. bilateral	Twice, double
Brady e.g. bradycardia	Slow
Bronch e.g. bronchitis	Bronchus, in the lungs
Cardio e.g. cardiomyopathy	Heart
Co e.g. comorbidity	With, together, in association with
Derm/derma/dermato e.g. dermatology	Skin
Di e.g. dissect	Separation, taking apart
Dys e.g. dysphagia	Bad, difficult
Gastro e.g. gastroenteritis	Stomach, belly
Haem e.g. haematology	Blood
Hyper e.g. hyperactive	Above, excessive
Hypo e.g. hypoactive	Below, deficient
Ophthalm(o) e.g. ophthalmology	Eye
Pharmaco e.g. pharmacology	Drug, medicine
Phleb(o) e.g. phlebotomy	Vein

Pneum(o) e.g. pneumothorax	Air, gas, lung, breathing
Poly e.g. polycystic	Many, multiple
Tachy e.g. tachycardia	Rapid
Therm(o) e.g. thermostatic	Heat
Thora/thorac(i) e.g. thoracentesis	Chest, thorax
Uni e.g. unilateral	One, single

INTRODUCTION AND GENERAL CONSIDERATIONS

FIONA EVERETT AND WENDY WRIGHT

Introduction

This book follows on from the *Essential Clinical Skills for Nurses: Step by Step*, 2nd edition (Delves-Yates, 2018) and therefore replicates many of the features contained within this book. It also accompanies the *Essentials of Nursing Adults* (Elcock et al., 2018). It has been written for nursing students undertaking a degree but can also serve as a useful resource for Health Care Support Workers (HCSW) and qualified practitioners.

This book has been developed by a dedicated team of lecturers who are actively engaged in teaching skills. They therefore recognise how important it is to master a skill in order to ensure that patients receive good quality care. Your exposure to different clinical skills may happen at different points on your journey to becoming a nurse. This will usually involve understanding the theory, learning through observation and active participation in a variety of clinical simulation experiences and clinical environments supported by a lecturer/supervisor/assessor.

However, it is important that you realise that the Nursing and Midwifery Council (NMC) *Standards for Proficiency for Registered Nurses* (NMC, 2018a), *Education Framework: Standards for Education and Training* (NMC, 2018b) and *Requirements for Pre-registration Nursing Education Programmes* (NMC, 2018c) set specific educational standards, which outline how nursing students must be educated and the proficiencies and skills that you must be able to demonstrate and attain in order to deliver and manage the current and future health needs of the population. Ultimately, the NMC require that you demonstrate attainment of the required level of knowledge and skills at the point of professional registration. The format and content of this book are therefore designed to support you to gain knowledge and skills, which are explained in a useful step by step approach with a rationale for each step.

Furthermore, this book presents you with information relating to each skill utilising a specific and consistent format as follows:

☑ **Before you start**

☑ **Essential equipment**

☑ **Care-setting considerations**

☑ **What to watch out for and action to take**

☑ **Helpful hints**

☑ **A step by step approach and the rationale for them**

Sources of information

A useful reference list has also been included, which will point you to further reading. Additional resources include:

- common abbreviations and useful prefixes and suffixes
- commonly used medication and side effects
- normal laboratory values
- hand-washing technique.

General considerations

Professionalism

The NMC is the UK regulator for the nursing and midwifery professions, whose aim is to serve the public by safeguarding their health and well-being. It achieves this by stipulating the personal and professional conduct expected from students and registered practitioners through the Code (NMC, 2018). The Code therefore ascertains the standards, which you must adhere to at every point of your journey to becoming a nurse and following registration.

The Code (NMC, 2018) identifies four key principles, which you must uphold. In doing so, you will demonstrate professionalism. These principles are as follows:

- prioritise people
- practice effectively
- preserve safety
- promote professionalism and trust.

Demonstrating professionalism is therefore a requirement in both your personal and professional life: this encompasses all environments and activities that you are engaged in. Performing clinical skills as part of person-centred good quality care is one aspect of your role, which can contribute to meeting the health needs of not only the individual but also the wider population. Furthermore, effective communication is also a requirement that will enable you to engage with patients and to gain their consent.

Gaining informed consent

Gaining informed consent prior to performing any skill or procedure is integral to the role of a nurse. However, this should be accompanied by a full and clear explanation, which will enable the patient to make an informed decision as to whether or not they wish to provide their consent.

It is therefore important to be mindful of an individual's level of understanding, so that consent and cooperation for the procedure can be gained. Allowing enough time for a full and clear explanation of what you are intending to do can support the patient to make a decision. You must also ensure that your knowledge and understanding in relation to mental capacity enables you to support the patient in their best interests. If a patient withholds their consent you may need to refer to local policies on presumed or assumed consent, which will mirror the stipulations of the Mental Capacity Act 2005 and best interest.

You will therefore be prompted in the step by step guide for each clinical procedure:

Before commencing any care activity, introduce yourself to the patient, explain the procedure and gain their consent

An accompanying rationale will be provided.

Infection prevention and control

Hand-washing is an essential clinical skill, which you will have been taught and practised numerous times. It is also a skill that is essential in the delivery of good quality patient-centred care. You will already be aware of the different types of hand-washing, the need for hand-washing to be performed and the different types of solutions which may be used. However, it is also important that you are aware of the relevant policy in relation to infection prevention and control.

You should also recognise the need to use appropriate personal protective equipment (PPE). This need is based on a robust risk assessment of the clinical procedure before you start.

You will therefore be prompted **appropriately** in the step by step guide for each clinical procedure:

> **Perform hand hygiene and apply non-sterile gloves only if required**
>
> **Apply sterile or non-sterile gloves as required**
>
> **Discard PPE, any single-use equipment and other used materials as per policy**

An accompanying rationale will be provided.

☑ Before you start

The 'before you start' step by step section sets out some of the common practices you will need to carry out at the start of a procedure, including things like:

> **Introducing yourself to the patient, explaining the procedure and gaining their consent**
>
> **Gathering the required equipment and ensuring it is as clean as appropriate and in working order**
>
> **Clear sufficient space within the environment, for example around the bed space or chair**
>
> **Wash your hands with soap and water before you start any care activity. Apron and gloves should only be worn if appropriate**

Ensure you promote patient dignity and privacy as appropriate, for example by drawing curtains

Patients need to be in a comfortable position

After performing the task, ensure the patient is in a comfortable position, with drinks and call bells available as necessary

Discard PPE, any single-use equipment and other used materials as per policy. Clean any equipment used as per the relevant policy every time it is used and perform hand hygiene

Document findings as appropriate, for example on the patient's observation chart and/or in the patient's notes

If any abnormalities are observed, escalate to senior nursing staff

An accompanying rationale will be provided.

☑ Essential equipment

The required 'essential equipment' will be recommended relevant to the clinical skill to be performed.

☑ Care-setting considerations

The clinical skills covered within this book can be performed in a variety of care settings. However, forward planning on your part will help you to ensure that the patient receives a good quality of care. Hand-washing is an example that can be used to illustrate the variation between care settings. If you are working in the patient's own home it is sensible to be prepared for a lack of running water, soap and clean hand towels. You can mitigate this by carrying your own supply of hand towels or hand wipes and always carry a hand sanitiser for situations when this is appropriate. However, ensuring that your hands are free from transient micro-organisms is an essential consideration irrespective of the care setting.

Another consideration is time appropriateness: if you are required to perform venepuncture (see Venepuncture chapter), for example, the quality of the specimen may be affected by the time of collection and the length of time before it reaches the laboratory. Again, if you are working in the patient's own home you would be required to have a knowledge of local policy, laboratory uplift schedules and recommended transportation and storage requirements to ensure safety and maintain the quality of the specimen.

The complexity of a procedure should also be considered to ensure that you have all the necessary equipment required and the support of another staff member who may be needed to assist and/or supervise the clinical skill being performed.

☑ What to watch out for and action to take

The 'what to watch out for and action to take' are common to a wide range of clinical skills. You will therefore notice the following information is standardised and recurs throughout the book:

> **While undertaking a clinical skill, you should also assess:**
>
> **The general condition of the patient: specific elements will vary according to the procedure being undertaken**
>
> **Their neurological condition - are they alert and responsive?**
>
> **Are they agitated?**
>
> **Any signs or complaints of pain or discomfort**
>
> **The patient's or relatives'/carers' views - for example, saying that their condition is 'not quite right' or they 'don't feel well'**

☑ Helpful hints

The helpful hints provide useful information when undertaking that particular skill; however, some are common to a wide range of clinical skills. You will therefore notice that the following information is standardised and recurs throughout this book:

> **Gloves and aprons must be worn if contact with blood/body fluids/excreta is anticipated or the patient is in isolation**

Hand hygiene must be performed before touching a patient, before clean/aseptic procedures, after body fluid exposure/ risk, after touching a patient and after touching a patient's surroundings

Waste products should be disposed of in a clinical waste bag if it is contaminated with blood/body fluids/excreta.

Sources of information will accompany the step by step approaches, which reflects evidence-based practice.

Source: Delves-Yates (2018); Elcock et al. (2018); NMC (2018, 2018a, 2018b, 2018c)

A note on terminology

The term 'patient' will be used throughout this book to refer to any person who receives any form of care.

References

Delves-Yates, C. (ed.) (2018) *Essential Clinical Skills for Nurses: Step By Step*, 2nd edn. London: Sage.

Elcock, K., Wright, W., Newcombe, P., Everett, F., (2018) *Essentials of Nursing Adults*. London: Sage.

Mental Capacity Act (2005) Available at: www.legislation.gov.uk/ ukpga/2005/9/pdfs/ukpga_20050009_en.pdf (accessed 10 August 2018).

Nursing and Midwifery Council (NMC) (2018) *The Code: Professional Standards of Practice and Behaviour for Nurses, Midwives and Nursing Associates*. London: NMC. Available at: www.nmc.org.uk/ globalassets/sitedocuments/nmc-publications/nmc-code.pdf (accessed 16 December 2018).

Nursing and Midwifery Council (NMC) (2018a) *Standards for Proficiency for Registered Nurses*. London: NMC.

Nursing and Midwifery Council (NMC) (2018b) *Education Framework: Standards for Education and Training*. London: NMC.

Nursing and Midwifery Council (NMC) (2018c) *Requirements for Pre-registration Nursing Education Programmes*. London: NMC.

BASIC AIRWAY MANAGEMENT
SOPHIE NEWCOMBE

☑ What is normal?

Most patients' airways will be patent. However, conditions such as reduced consciousness, foreign bodies, anaphylaxis, facial trauma or infection, burns and tumours can cause partial or complete airway obstruction. Airway obstruction can be insidious or quick. Nurses should monitor and assess the airway regularly and quickly escalate any concerns to the medical team.

☑ Before you start

This chapter follows the Resuscitation Council (UK) 2015 guidelines.

☑ Essential equipment

Basic airway equipment, available in all care settings, should include:

- suction (portable or wall mounted) with rigid (Yankauer) and soft suction catheters
- oropharyngeal airways (OPA), sizes 2-4
- nasopharyngeal airways (NPA), sizes 6-8.

☑ Field-specific considerations

A patient with learning disabilities could have reduced cognition which will necessitate a different approach to informed consent and time taken to explain procedures. This might also be true for paediatrics. Additionally parents and carers need to be included in their care. Babies and children, because of the different anatomy and physiology, will require smaller equipment and insertion techniques can vary depending on age. Please refer to appropriate guidelines for further information.

Patients who have mental health problems or those with a reduced level of understanding might withhold consent. Furthermore, some of the procedures within this chapter will be performed because the patient has deteriorated and it is an emergency situation. Thus sometimes consent cannot be obtained and procedures are done in the patient's best interest. Please refer to the Mental Capacity Act 2005.

Airway assessment

Airway comes first in the ABCDE approach to patient assessment and management. This ensures the most significant threat to life is recognised and treated first.

Initial assessment is easily achieved by talking to your patient. Ask a simple open-ended question like 'How are you feeling?' A verbal response indicates that their airway is patent. If the patient does not respond verbally (in the absence of known aphasia), assume that the airway is not patent and at risk. Check for a response immediately. Gently shake their shoulders and give a command loudly in both ears, such as 'Open your eyes'. No response - call for help/use the emergency bell.

- **Look**
  Normal breathing is effortless. Look at their work of breathing. Check for use of accessory muscles in the neck, nasal flaring, lip pursing or tracheal tug. Ensure the trachea is central. Expose their chest (maintaining privacy and dignity); look for symmetry of breathing and intercostal recession, peripheral or central cyanosis.

- **Listen**
  Normal breath sounds are quiet. Listen for sounds. Noises indicating a partial upper airway obstruction include gurgling, (due to secretions, vomit or blood), snoring (a result of flaccid muscles around the oropharynx) and stridor.

- **Feel**
  Feel for breath at the mouth and nose.

Manoeuvres - head tilt/chin lift: step by step

If the patient's airway is compromised take immediate action to relieve the obstruction and maintain a patent airway. An obstructed airway will lead to respiratory arrest and potentially death. This manoeuvre relieves upper airway obstruction:

 With the patient supine, place one hand (palm down) on their forehead
To stabilise the head

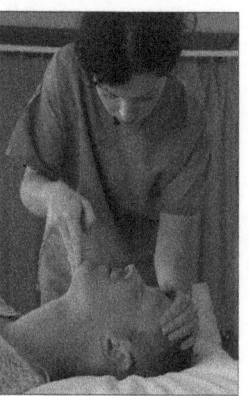

Place two/three fingers under the bony point of their chin
To avoid damaging the soft tissues and reduce the risk of further airway obstruction

Tilt their head gently backwards whilst applying upwards pressure with your fingers under the chin
To relieve obstruction by lifting the anterior neck structures

Manoeuvres - jaw thrust: step by step

An alternative manoeuvre which should be used if cervical spine injury is suspected:

 With the patient supine, identify the patient's angle of the jaw. Place your fingers under the angle of the jaw on either side
To identify the landmarks and correctly locate the mandible

Once your fingers are in place, apply steady upwards and forward pressure
To lift the jaw vertically and open the airway

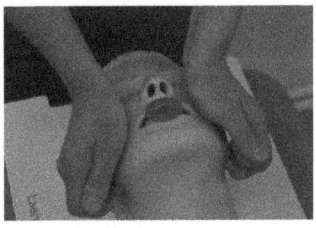

 Using your thumbs, slightly open the mouth by downward displacement of the chin
To bring the mandible forward thus relieving obstruction by the tongue, soft palate and epiglottis

Airway adjuncts

Adjuncts are helpful in maintaining an airway. Head tilt or jaw thrust may still be required, however.

Oropharyngeal airway (OPA): step by step

The OPA lifts the tongue away from the oropharynx. It is a hard curved plastic tube, flanged and reinforced at the end. Use only in unconscious patients or respiratory/cardiac arrest, due to the risk of vomiting or laryngospasm if the patient's gag reflex is present.

 Wash your hands and put on clean gloves
To minimise cross infection

 With the patient supine measure the OPA from the angle of their jaw to the level of their incisors
To estimate the size of OPA required

 Open the patient's mouth. Use a Yankauer sucker to quickly clear any vomit, blood or secretions if necessary
To avoid secretions blocking the OPA or being pushed further down during insertion

4 Insert the OPA upside down into the oral cavity, so that the end points up towards the hard palate. Keep the OPA upside down and advance it into the mouth
The OPA's convex shape depresses the tongue and reduces the risk of pushing the tongue back as it is advanced

5 Once the OPA is at the junction of the hard and soft palate, rotate it 180 degrees
To avoid trauma to the soft palate

6 Continue to advance the OPA until it lies within the pharynx and the flange rests at the lips
To secure a patent airway

7 Check patency and breathing by using the look, listen, feel technique
To ensure that the intervention has been effective

8 Remove the OPA if the patient coughs, strains or gags
The OPA could cause vomiting or laryngospasm if gag reflex is present

9 Remove gloves and wash your hands
In accordance with infection control precautions

10 Reassess and closely monitor patient. A patient with an OPA in situ should not be left unattended
The patient can quickly deteriorate

Nasopharyngeal airway (NPA): step by step

The NPA creates an airway via the nasopharynx. It is a soft malleable tube which has a flange at one end and is bevelled at the other. The NPA can be used in patients with an intact gag reflex, trismus or oral trauma. It is contraindicated in coagulopathy and basal skull or nasal fractures.

1 Patients can be upright or supine for insertion. The NPA size is estimated based on patient size
Size 6 - small adult, size 8 - large adult

2 **Explain procedure and gain consent if applicable**
The patient might be conscious

3 **Wash your hands and put on clean gloves**
To minimise cross infection

4 **Apply a water-based lubricant to the NPA and insert bevel toward the nasal septum**
To aid insertion

5 **Advance horizontally, following the curvature of the nasopharyngeal cavity**
To minimise trauma

6 **Rotate 90 degrees so the NPA is in the nasopharynx and the tip is behind the uvula**
To secure a patent airway

7 **Check patency and breathing by using the look, listen, feel technique**
To ensure that the intervention has been effective

8 **Remove gloves and wash your hands**
In accordance with infection control precautions

☑ Helpful hints

- After each intervention reassess your patient to check it has worked.
- Jaw thrust can be tiring so swap if necessary.
- Remove any broken or displaced dentures but leave well-fitting dentures in place.
- OPA insertion is easier if you stand behind the patient's head.
- An OPA that is slightly too big is more beneficial than one that is too small.
- OPAs are colour coded but colours may vary depending on manufacturer.
- Some NPAs require a safety pin through the flange: ensure this is in place before insertion.
- Flexible suction is possible through OPA and NPA.

Recovery position

☑ Before you start

Ensure that it is safe to approach.

If the patient is breathing but their airway is compromised or at risk, they can be nursed (with or without an adjunct) in the recovery position. It should not be used unless absolutely necessary in patients with suspected spinal fractures.

☑ Field-specific considerations

A child under one would not be put into the recovery position. Instead they would be held, facing out with their head tilted downwards (so their face and airway is visible and secretions are able to freely drain).

☑ Care-setting considerations

The recovery position can be performed in any care setting either on on a bed/trolley or on the floor.

Using the recovery position: step by step

1 **Open the airway using either head tilt/chin lift or jaw thrust and ensure that the patient is breathing**
The recovery position should only be performed if the patient is breathing normally

2 **Quickly and safely remove any spectacles and/or sharp objects from the patient's pockets**
To prevent injury to patient

3 **Bend the arm nearest to you at the elbow with their hand pointing upwards to create a right angle**
To facilitate rolling the patient and prevent them from rolling onto the full length of their arm

4 **Bring their other arm across their chest with the back of their hand against their cheek. Place your palm against theirs**
To support their head

5 Bend the leg furthest from you at the knee, keeping their foot on the bed/floor
To facilitate rolling the patient

6 Pull on the bent leg so the patient rolls towards you onto their side
To facilitate rolling

7 Position the upper leg so that the hip and knee create a right angle
To 'anchor' the patient and prevent them from rolling forwards or backwards

8 Tilt the head back to open the airway. Use their palm to support their head and ensure their head is tilted downwards
To allow the tongue to fall forwards and promote drainage

9 Reassess and continue to closely monitor the patient. Get help if not already done
The patient might deteriorate

References

Mental Capacity Act (2005) Available at: www.legislation.gov.uk/ukpga/2005/9/pdfs/ukpga_20050009_en.pdf (accessed 10 August 2018).

Resuscitation Council (UK) (2015) *Resuscitation Guidelines* 2015. London: Resuscitation Council (UK).

ADVANCED AIRWAY MANAGEMENT

KAMALPREET KAUR DHINDSA

Rigid catheter suctioning

Oropharyngeal secretions can be removed with a wide-bore rigid sucker (Yankauer).

☑ Before you start

- Use with caution if the patient has an intact gag reflex.
- Essential safety checks should be done before beginning the procedure.

☑ Essential equipment

- Functioning suction unit (portable or wall-mounted depending on clinical setting)
- Connection tubing
- Rigid catheter (Yankauer)
- PPE non-sterile gloves (+ visor and apron if splashes are likely)
- Sterile bowl/jug
- Sterile water

☑ Field-specific considerations

Refer to your hospital policy when dealing with neonates and children.

☑ Care-setting considerations

Portable suction units may be used in out-of-hospital settings.

☑ What to watch out for and action to take

Rigid catheter suctioning is contraindicated in patients with suspected basal skull fractures.

☑ Helpful Hints

- Suction devices should be inspected at least daily.
- Saline nebulisers can be used in case of thick secretions.
- Perform a pre- and post-suction respiratory assessment to monitor for improvement.

Rigid catheter suctioning: step by step

(1) Explain procedure and gain consent if applicable
Where possible informed consent should be obtained to gain patient's cooperation and promote trust in healthcare professionals. Fully informed consent may not be possible in emergency situations, when dealing with children or people with learning disabilities or impaired mental capacity. Involve family and carers where possible

(2) Gather supplies
To avoid any unnecessary delays during the procedure

(3) Wash hands and put on clean gloves (consider additional PPE)
To prevent cross infection. Consider the need to wear protective eye gear to avoid any splashes

(4) Turn suction on to the required level (normally 100-150 mmHg/20 kPa)
To facilitate effective removal of secretions and minimise the possibility of trauma to the airway

(5) Test suction works by suctioning a small amount of the water
To ensure suction apparatus is in working condition before beginning the procedure

6 Position patient correctly: unconscious patients should be in a supine or lateral position and conscious patients should be in a semi-Fowler's position
Semi-Fowler's position facilitates ease of suctioning in conscious patients. Supine or lateral position prevents tongue from falling back and blocking the airways. Guedel airway should be used in unconscious patients

7 Remove oxygen mask if present. Nasal cannula can remain in situ
To facilitate effective removal of secretions

8 Insert Yankauer gently into mouth and apply suction (often achieved by covering the thumb hole on the catheter)
To avoid any trauma to the airway

9 Only suction as far as you can see and suction for no more than 10-15 seconds
To avoid hypoxia

10 Replace oxygen and allow patient to rest between suctioning if required
To avoid hypoxia

11 Clear catheter and tubing by suctioning a small amount of water
To facilitate the removal of any secretions from the suction catheter and prevent spread of infection

12 Reassess and repeat if required
To assess the need for repeat suctioning

13 Remove gloves and wash your hands
To adhere to infection control policies

14 Document
Document the amount, colour and consistency of the secretions

Endotracheal intubation

Intubation is the placement of an endotracheal tube in the trachea and is the gold standard method of choice for the establishment and maintenance of an airway. It may be performed as a planned procedure or as an emergency.

☑ Before you start

- Refer to trust guidelines for specific considerations.
- Vital signs, saturation levels and ECG should be monitored during the procedure.
- Suction and oxygen equipment should be checked and available.

☑ Essential equipment

- Laryngoscope handle and curved blades (additional spare blades, sizes 3-4)
- Cuffed endotracheal tubes (ETT), sizes 6.0-8.0 mm
- 10 ml syringe
- Stethoscope
- Waveform capnography
- Lubricating jelly
- Magill's forceps
- Introducers: bougie and stylet
- Tape/bandage
- Self-inflating bag with reservoir - bag-valve-mask (BVM)
- Suction unit with Yankauer and range of smaller flexible catheters
- IV drugs, if needed

☑ Field-specific considerations

During a planned procedure, people with learning difficulties might necessitate a different approach to informed consent so allow extra time to explain the procedure. The size of the ETT will vary when dealing with children. Refer to your hospital guidelines for further information.

☑ Care-setting considerations

Endotracheal intubations are performed in highly specialised areas liked critical care or in theatres. Emergency, out-of-hospital intubation is usually performed by specially trained paramedics and doctors.

☑ What to watch out for and action to take

Patients should be observed very carefully for any signs of respiratory distress during suctioning. Any signs of respiratory distress should be reported promptly.

- Check the cuff, pilot balloon and valve of ETT prior to use.
- Check for patent IV access.
- Ensure suction apparatus is working.
- Procedure should be limited to maximum of 15-20 seconds.

Endotracheal intubation: step by step

(1) **Where possible, explain the procedure to the patient and obtain informed consent**
Informed consent, where possible, should be obtained to gain the patient's cooperation and to promote trust

(2) **Gather equipment**
To avoid any unnecessary delays during the procedure

(3) **The patient should be supine with bed head removed. Place the pillow under the head and extend the neck**
To open the airway and facilitate better visualisation of the vocal cords during intubation

(4) **The anaesthetist will manually ventilate the patient with 100% oxygen, using a BVM prior to intubation**
Manual ventilation is undertaken to prevent hypoxia during the procedure

(5) **Anaesthetic drugs (induction agents and muscles relaxants) are administered, if required**
In the conscious patient, this will allow relaxation of the protective airway reflexes, but also cause cessation of breathing. This is not usually required in situations such as cardiac arrest

(6) **Consider applying cricoid pressure to minimise passive regurgitation and aspiration of gastric contents**
The cricoid cartilage is located immediately below the thyroid cartilage and forms a complete ring at the upper end of the trachea

(7) **When the anaesthetist can visualise the glottis using a laryngoscope, the ETT is inserted whilst the vocal cords**

are open, until the vocal cord guide is at the level of the vocal cords (black ring around the tip of the tube)
It is essential the ETT is passed into the trachea and not the oesophagus. Also, the correct length will avoid intubation of the right or left main bronchus

(8) Inflate the cuff to optimal pressure (25-30 cm H_2O)
Cuff inflation creates a secure seal and also prevents dislodgement of the tube

(9) Confirm correct tube placement
Primary assessment of correct tube placement includes bilateral chest expansion and auscultation over the lung field. The gold standard for correct tube placement confirmation is end-tidal CO_2 detectors that include a waveform graphic display

(10) Connect ETT (via a catheter mount) to the ventilating device
This will allow the patient to breathe via oxygen-enriched ventilation

(11) Secure the ETT with a tie
To prevent dislodgement of the tube

(12) Observe the patient's vital signs during the procedure, notifying the team of any changes
To facilitate patient assessment during the procedure and note any deviation from baseline

(13) The procedure should be stopped if the patient deteriorates, i.e. bradycardia, desaturation
To avoid deterioration. BVM ventilation with 100% oxygen should occur immediately

Tracheostomy care - dressing change

Tracheostomy dressings should be changed at least daily or when wet because of secretions. It is a two-person technique.

☑ **Before you start**

Check your trust policies and guidelines with regards to suctioning and dressing changes.

☑ **Equipment needed**

- PPE eye protection
- Suction equipment
- Emergency intubation kit in case of accidental decannulation
- A tracheostomy dressing and tapes/ties
- Sterile dressing pack with gauze
- Normal saline or sterile water
- A swab and specimen container

☑ **Field-specific considerations**

An assistant may be required to help support the patient where cognitive impairment exists. Appropriate dressing sizes are available for neonates and children.

☑ **Care-setting considerations**

Dressing changes may be performed in hospital or community settings.

☑ **Helpful hints**

- Gather all the equipment beforehand.
- Assess your patient's vital signs and respiratory function as a baseline before beginning procedure.
- Assess the need to suction before beginning procedure.

Tracheostomy care - dressing change: step by step

1 **Explain the procedure to the patient, gain informed consent**
Where possible, informed consent should be obtained to gain patient's cooperation and promote trust

2 Position the patient so the stoma and tracheostomy tube are clearly visible
Good positioning enhances visibility and prevents accidental dislodgement of the tracheostomy tube.

3 Wash hands and put on PPE
To prevent cross infection

4 Open dressing pack, tracheostomy dressing and tapes/ties onto dressing trolley using an aseptic non-touch technique (ANTT)
To ensure correct equipment is easily accessible and sterility is maintained

5 Instruct assistant to hold the tracheostomy tube securely in position
To prevent dislodgement of the tracheostomy tube during dressing change

6 Remove the old dressing and tapes and inspect the stoma for any signs of infection. If signs of infection are noted, take a swab for microscopy
Look for any redness, swelling or break in skin integrity around the stoma

7 Clean around the stoma with gauze and sterile water
To minimise infection

8 Inspect the stoma and skin around for any redness and swelling, use barrier cream if needed
To prevent pressure sores

9 Apply the sterile tracheostomy dressing around the stoma and tracheostomy tube
To minimise infection and prevent pressure sores

10 Attach the new tracheostomy tapes. Ensure tapes are not too tight by checking that one or two fingers can be inserted between the tapes and the patient's neck
To prevent pressure sores

11 Check the cuff pressure (20-24 cm H_2O)
Optimal cuff pressure should be maintained all the time to prevent any dislodgement

Dispose of the dressing and other equipment used and wash your hands
To prevent cross infection. Dressing should be disposed of as per hospital policy

 Reassess your patient to identify changes in vital signs
Look for any signs of respiratory distress and changes in vital signs

 Document
Document the time of dressing change in patient's note. Any changes in skin or signs of infection should be documented clearly and reported as per trust policy

Source: Dougherty and Lister (2015); Merriman (2017)

References

Dougherty, L. and Lister, S.E. (eds) (2015) *The Royal Marsden Manual of Clinical Nursing Procedures*, 9th edn. Chichester: Wiley-Blackwell.

LUNG SOUNDS

KAMALPREET KAUR DHINDSA

Auscultation

☑ What is normal?

Lungs sounds are the noises made as air moves through the small and large airways during inspiration and expiration. Auscultation is the process used to listen to lung sounds with a stethoscope. Familiarity with normal lung sounds allows the identification of abnormal lung sounds and facilitates consideration of the underlying causes.

- **Vesicular:** These are quiet, low-pitched sounds. There is no pause between inspiration and expiration. Expiration is longer than inspiration. Vesicular breath sounds are heard in the peripheries of the lung.
- **Bronchial:** These are loud, high-pitched sounds. There is no pause between inspiration and expiration. Inspiration equals expiration. Bronchial breath sounds are heard over the trachea.
- **Bronchovesicular:** These are a combination of the above sounds, heard over the major airways and most parts of the lungs.

☑ Before you start

- Obtain informed consent and ensure your patient understands the process.
- Position your patient comfortably, usually upright or sitting.
- Ideally auscultation should be conducted in a quiet environment.

- Diaphragm of the stethoscope
- Sterets to clean ear plugs before and after use
- Hand-washing facilities or alcohol rub for hand disinfection

☑ **Field-specific considerations**

In those with cognitive impairment, it is important to ascertain the patient's level of understanding when gaining consent. Involve the family when dealing with children. Use a paediatric stethoscope for babies and smaller children.

☑ **Care-setting considerations**

Auscultation can be undertaken in any setting where privacy can be maintained.

☑ **What to watch out for and action to take**

There are a range of abnormal or adventitious (added) lung sounds which generally indicate underlying pathophysiology.

Musical sounds

a. **Stridor** - musical, high-pitched sounds heard over the upper airways. May be audible without a stethoscope. Indicates upper airway obstruction.
b. **Wheeze** - musical high-pitched sounds heard on inspiration or expiration or both. Can be localised or generalised. Caused by airway narrowing or blockage.

Non-musical sounds

a. **Fine crackles** - non-musical, short and explosive sounds heard on mid to late inspiration and occasionally on expiration. Unaffected by cough. Associated with various lung diseases, e.g. pulmonary fibrosis, congestive heart failure or pneumonia. Not associated with secretions.
b. **Coarse crackles** - non-musical, short sounds heard on early inspiration and throughout expiration, affected by cough. Indicate intermittent airway opening, related to secretions.

c. **Pleural friction rub** - sounds which are creaking in nature, typically heard over basal regions. Heard more clearly on deep breathing. Associated with pleural inflammation.

☑ Helpful hints

Use the diaphragm of the stethoscope to listen to the lungs in the following systematic manner:

- **Posterior chest:** auscultate from side to side and top to bottom. Consider starting at the base for patients with breathlessness.
- **Anterior chest:** auscultate from side to side and top to bottom in between first to seventh intercostal spaces.
- **Lateral chest:** auscultate from top to bottom over the underlying lobe.

Compare one side with other and listen for symmetry. Document the location and quality of sounds heard.

Auscultation: step by step

(1) **Introduce yourself and gain informed consent**
To gain the patient's trust and their cooperation during the procedure

(2) **Gather all the equipment needed and ensure it is clean and in working order**
To avoid any unnecessary delays and reduce the risk of infection

(3) **Position yourself optimally, avoiding bending or twisting over the patient and, where possible, conduct the assessment in a quiet environment.**
To promote audibility and minimise risk of back injury

(4) **Remove only essential clothing as briefly as possible and ensure doors/curtains are closed**
To maintain patient's dignity and privacy during the procedure

5 Wash your hands before beginning the procedure. Wear aprons, gloves and face masks where needed
PPE used based on individual patient's risk of infection

6 Position your patient comfortably, ideally sitting or upright position
Allows full lung expansion

7 Ask the patient to take deep breaths through the mouth
Enhances the audibility of lung sounds

8 Using the stethoscope, auscultate the lungs in a stepwise manner (as mentioned above)
Ensures thorough assessment and facilitates comparison between different lung fields

9 Replace clothing and reposition patient
To promote dignity and comfort

10 Document findings in the patient's notes and escalate any concerns based on the findings
Ensures accurate record keeping and facilitates decision-making

References

Bohadana, A., Izbicki, G. and Kraman, S.S. (2015) 'Fundamentals of lung auscultation', *The New England Journal of Medicine, 370*(8): 744-51.

OXYGEN THERAPY
KAREN ELLIOTT

☑ Before you start

Oxygen must be prescribed as a drug, so ensure you check the following:

- ensure a correct prescription is available for oxygen specifically for the patient
- check the patient identification and obtain informed consent
- ensure patient's understanding of the oxygen therapy
- target oxygen saturation levels are set for the respective patient.*

*The British Thoracic Society (BTS) recommendation is to achieve a target saturation of 94-98% for the most acutely ill patients or 88-92%, or the patient's normal target range for those at risk of hypercapnic respiratory failure. Refer to *Titrating Oxygen Up and Down Using the Mask Escalator* (BTS, 2017b) for guidance.

☑ Essential equipment

- Oxygen supply (central or cylinder)
- Appropriate delivery device (see chart below)
- Oxygen tubing
- A humidifier - warm water- or cold water-based systems *for humidified oxygen therapy only*
- T-piece connector, for use with tracheostomy tubes (if not delivering via a mask) *for humidified oxygen therapy only*

☑ Field-specific considerations

Oxygen delivery devices can be claustrophobic, so people with cognitive impairment or those who are anxious may need extra reassurance and support to enable safe and effective oxygen administration. Smaller size devices are available for children.

☑ Care-setting considerations

In hospital, piped gases will be available, whereas in the community oxygen cylinders are more likely; consider the safe moving and handling of oxygen cylinders.

Health and safety - oxygen is a combustible gas. Care must be taken with activities and products that exacerbate this, i.e. smoking, Vaseline, hand creams, alcohol-based products (MRHA, 2012)

☑ What to watch out for and action to take

Oxygen should be administered and delivered according to the patient's prescription: there is a wide range of delivery devices which can be classified into low and high flow oxygen devices. Selection is made on the basis of a patient's SpO_2 levels and underlying condition. Table 1 is a guide as to possible choices and delivery considerations.

☑ Helpful hints

- For patients at risk of type 2 respiratory failure, target saturation levels should be 88-92%. Start off with a fixed flow (Venturi mask), ideally blue or white, maintaining saturation levels at 88-92%.
- For patients not at risk of type 2 respiratory failure, maintain SpO_2 levels at 94-98%. For initial hypoxaemia (SpO_2 less than 85%) use non-rebreather mask. For SpO_2 levels of 85-94%, start with nasal cannula at 2-6 L/min or simple face mask at 5-10 L/min and titrate accordingly.
- When patients are receiving oxygen therapy, ongoing assessment should be followed in line with local policy. This might include: assessment and observation of the patient's general condition, i.e. breathing rate, pattern, sounds, position, use of accessory muscles as well as ongoing assessment with NEWS2, including respiratory rate, SpO_2 monitoring.
- Blood gas monitoring could be required if clinically indicated.
- Oral hygiene and dryness of the mouth and lips; encourage patients to sip water regularly or assist with mouthcare if required.

Table 1 Oxygen delivery systems

Oxygen delivery device	Flow rate (L/min)	FiO$_2$ (approx.) & % equivalent	Specific considerations
Nasal cannula	1-6	0.24-0.44 24%-44%	More comfortable for the patients Prolonged use can lead to dryness of mucosa
Simple face mask	5-8	0.40-0.60 40%-60%	Minimum flow rate of 5L/min to prevent rebreathing and accumulation of CO$_2$
Non-rebreathing mask	10-15	0.90-1.00 90%-100%	Attached reservoir bag to provide additional volume Used in critically ill patients requiring high levels of supplemental oxygen

(Continued)

Table 1 (Continued)

Oxygen delivery device	Flow rate (L/min)	FiO$_2$ (approx.) & % equivalent	Specific considerations
Venturi mask	2-15	0.24-0.60 24%-60%	Exact FiO$_2$ can be delivered
			Comes with colour coded attachments that deliver specific FiO$_2$ levels
			Blue - 24% - 2L White - 28% - 4L Yellow - 35% - 8L Red - 40% - 10L Green - 60% - 15L
Humidified oxygen system	2-15	0.24-0.60 24%-60%	Most humidified oxygen systems use a Venturi delivery system. See the box above for guidance.
			Humidified oxygen delivery is beneficial to patients with artificial airways, such as tracheostomy, or to prevent dryness and assist with sputum clearance (BTS, 2017a).

- Irritation to eyes – this can be caused by ill-fitting face masks: check the mask chosen fits and moulds to the patient's face.
- Check skin integrity regularly observing areas around ears, nose and mouth for any soreness, redness, cracking of the skin that devices or oxygen might be causing.
- Humidified oxygen therapy systems can be noisy; consider the setting and possible disruptions to the patient and others.

Oxygen therapy: step by step

1 **Collect the required equipment and patient prescription**
Ensure that the appropriate documentation trail is evident and oxygen is correctly prescribed specifically for the patient. Refer to local policy and medicine administration guidelines. Refer to the text and table above to assist in selecting the most appropriate equipment required

2 **Confirm the patient identity and consent for oxygen therapy**
Informed consent requires the patient to be given insight into the pros and cons of receiving oxygen therapy. This aids patient understanding and compliance in the delivery of treatment and hopefully reduces any related anxieties

Not all patients will be fit to consent to oxygen therapy; in these situations seek help and advice from a qualified health care practitioner to open discussion, but in the case of emergencies oxygen can be administered without a prescription (BTS, 2017a)

3 **Assist and make the patient comfortable ideally in an upright supported sitting position**
A sitting position is favourable as this will allow for effective lung expansion and breathing. However, any positioning must be suitable and adapted to each individual patient for optimum comfort

4 **Effectively decontaminate hands then assemble the required clean equipment; attach the oxygen delivery device to the tubing as required**
New, clean equipment should be opened and used for every patient, to prevent the risk of cross infection. Refer to the

equipment manufacturer's instructions as required. Ensure sufficient tubing is selected/cut to allow for the distance between the patient and the oxygen source, plus allowing for additional movement the patient may require in and around the care environment

5 **Connect the assembled device and tubing directly to the oxygen flow meter outlet**
The far end of the tubing will be connected to the flow meter outlet. Check and ensure that the flow meter being used is delivering the required gas: oxygen. This can be confused especially if there is a twin flow meter. Ensure the connections are secure to avoid leaking/escaping of oxygen

6 **Apply the chosen delivery mask or device to the patient's face**
Fit the mask or nasal specs to the patient, ensuring a good fit around the mouth and nose. This will prevent escaping oxygen and ensure accurate delivery. This step is important to prevent complications with eyes and skin integrity which can be caused by poor-fitting delivery devices. If comfort is considered it should assist with compliance in the wearing and tolerance of the therapy

7 **Switch on the oxygen and set the flow meter to the required rate**
Open the flow meter to move the ball/bobbin to the required flow rate. This is indicated by the centre of the floating ball being aligned with the appropriate flow rate number/marking. Alignment is essential for ensuring the accuracy of delivery (BTS, 2017a)

8 **Humidified oxygen therapy**
Ensure that the tubing is kept below the height of the mask to prevent any possible back flow of water: the tube should be checked at regular intervals to empty any condensed water from the tubing as this could pose an infection risk if left

9 **Monitor the patient and response to therapy as required**
Ongoing monitoring is essential to ensure safe and effective oxygen administration and will be dictated by the patient's condition and local policy

Source: All photos are original photos taken by the Author; Karen Elliott

References

British Thoracic Society (BTS) (2017a) 'Guidelines of the use of oxygen in adults in healthcare and emergency settings', *Thorax*, *72*(Supp1): i1-i90.

British Thoracic Society (BTS) (2017b) *Titrating Oxygen Up and Down Using the Mask Escalator*. Available at: https://slideplayer.com/slide/12272267/ (accessed 5 October 2018).

Medicines and Healthcare Products Regulatory Agency (MHRA) (2012) *Medical Oxygen, 100% Medical Gas Compressed PL27970/0001*. Cheshire: CSTS Ltd.

NEBULISERS

KAREN ELLIOTT

Nebulised therapy is frequently used for patients with severe asthma and COPD. All nebuliser therapy must be prescribed including the required driving gas for the nebuliser to be administered; this will be oxygen or air, dependent on the patient's condition (BTS, 2017a).

Nebulisers are a form of drug administration/therapy used to deliver a liquid drug via a fine cloud-like mist for inspiration into the respiratory tract. Drugs that are commonly nebulised include: bronchodilators, glucocorticosteroids, normal saline (0.9% sodium chloride) and possibly antibiotics.

☑ Before you start

- Check the patient's prescription, identification and allergies.
- Ensure the patient's consent and understanding of nebulised therapy.
- Ensure an appropriate delivery device is chosen, dependent on patient needs; consider age, manual dexterity, strength, coordination (Rogliani et al., 2017).
- Ensure the patient is in an upright position allowing for chest expansion.

☑ Essential equipment

- Driving gas - this could be piped/cylinder oxygen/air or an air compressor
- Nebuliser delivery set - including mask or mouthpiece dependent on patient's need
- Tubing
- Solution/drug to be administered as prescribed

☑ Field-specific considerations

See section on Oxygen Therapy. Appropriate doses will be required in children.

☑ Care-setting considerations

In hospital it is probable that piped gases will be available, whereas in the community air compressors or oxygen cylinders are more likely. Ensure the patient is aware and taught how to set up, clean and store the equipment required when in a community setting.

☑ Helpful hints

- Patients with asthma will generally be prescribed oxygen – the driving gas for nebuliser therapy.
- Consider eye conditions if using a mask for delivery, as masks can allow leakage of mist up into the eyes – a mouthpiece is preferable.
- Consider if peak flow measurements are required pre- and post-nebuliser to monitor for treatment effectiveness.
- All equipment, air compressors, nebuliser sets, should be used and cleaned in accordance with the manufacturer instructions/guidance and local policy.
- Assess the patient for the most suitable delivery device; consider the point above when making a decision between mask or mouthpiece.
- If the patient is able, ask them to tap the sides of the nebuliser chamber to release droplets that have been aerated and stuck to the side walls. This can aid the full dose of medication to be administered.

Nebulised therapy: step by step

(1) **Assemble the required equipment including the prescription and drug to be used**
Following assessment, collect a clean, suitable delivery device, mask or mouthpiece set along with the drug ampoule in accordance with the appropriate medication policy, procedures and checks

2 **Confirm patient's identity and consent to proceed**
In accordance with medication policy and procedures, confirm you have the correct patient. Discuss the treatment to be given ensuring the patient understands and agrees to the nebulised drug therapy. Informed consent requires the patient to be given insight into the pros and cons of receiving therapy. This aids the patient's understanding and compliance in the delivery of treatment and hopefully reduces any related anxieties

3 **Assist and make patient comfortable in an upright sitting position if able and confirm suitability for using chosen delivery set (mask/mouthpiece)**
Nebuliser therapy can take 10-20 minutes to administer so it is important that the patient is comfortable, ideally in an upright position to enable good breathing and lung expansion. Confirm that the patient can hold the mouthpiece in place for the duration of treatment or consider the use of a mask which can be held in place with a strap allowing the patient to relax their arms

4 **Record and document pre peak flow measurement if required**
Instruct the patient to undertake a peak flow measurement if clinically able to and required: this may assist with the monitoring of the effectiveness of treatment. Document recordings on a peak flow measurement chart

5 **Check drug against the prescription in accordance with local policy for medicine administration**
Before administering the drug via the nebuliser, complete the checks as required, considering: right drug, dose, time, patient, route in line with local policy and medication procedures

6 **Decontaminate your hands and assemble mask/ mouthpiece with the nebuliser chamber**
In accordance with infection control policies ensure hands are clean when opening and assembling clean equipment and devices. Refer to the manufacturer instructions as required to assemble the set

Open the nebuliser chamber and pour in medication to one side (avoid pouring into the middle as this goes into the tubing). Once assembled unscrew the nebuliser chamber to remove the top, exposing the nebuliser chamber.
The medication to be nebulised should be poured into the chamber, avoiding the middle section which could cause spillage, reducing the drug dosage

 Screw on the nebuliser lid supporting the mask/ mouthpiece, attaching tubing to bottom of chamber Once the drug is added, re-attach the chamber lid securely.
Holding upright to avoid spillage, attach the tubing firmly to the bottom of the chamber

 Attach tubing to the prescribed gas flow meter/ compressor according to the prescription
Connect the far end of the tubing to the gas source - this could be oxygen or compressed air. Check the prescription chart to ensure correct delivery in line with medication policy and procedures

 Place the mask or mouthpiece on the patient and switch on driving gas source
The patient should be ready, mask on or mouthpiece in position before switching on the nebuliser; this allows for the full dosage to be received by the patient as prescribed. The gas if using a flow meter should be switched to approximately. 6-8 L/min or until the drug can be seen as a fine mist (BTS, 2017a)

 Advise breathing normally and no talking for the duration of the nebuliser
Encourage the patient to try and relax, taking normal breaths and expanding their chest fully. This allows for the drug to be inhaled fully into the lungs for maximum effect

 Once the liquid has all evaporated, turn off the gas and remove mask/mouthpiece
When the liquid has all evaporated and the chamber is empty the drug has been administered. Turn off of the driving gas source and remove the patient's mask/mouthpiece

(13) Document drug administered on the drug chart in accordance with local policy for medicine administration
Complete the documentation in line with medication policy and procedures. Note the time that the nebuliser was started to complete documentation

(14) Encourage patients to have a drink or mouthwash if there is an odd taste left
Encourage drinking afterwards to avoid an unpleasant taste or any residual drug left in the mouth

(15) Wash and dry the nebuliser chamber according to local policy, label clearly with the patient's name
All equipment is single patient use only so should be clearly stored, labelled and changed according to local policy

(16) Record and document post peak flow measurement if required
If a pre-treatment peak flow measurement was recorded then ideally a post-treatment/nebuliser measurement should also be taken around 15 minutes after the nebuliser was administered and documented on the peak flow chart to provide a comparison for monitoring effectiveness of treatment. A positive rise in post-treatment peak flows would be indicative of effective treatment

Source: Dunk and Talbot (2016)

References

British Thoracic Society (BTS) (2017a) `Guidelines of the use of oxygen in adults in healthcare and emergency settings', *Thorax*, 72(Supp1): i1 -i90.

Dunk, R. and Talbot, S. (2016) *Nebulisers*. Available at: www.clinical skills.net

Rogliani, P., Calzette, L., Coppola, A., Cavalli, F., Ora, J., Puxeddu, E., et al. (2017) 'Optimizing drug delivery in COPD: The role of inhaler devices', *Respiratory Medicine*, 124: 6-14.

VENEPUNCTURE

WINNIE MCGARRY AND CAROLINE MACCALLUM

☑ Before you start

Remember the common steps for all care delivered to assist patients. This procedure uses the aseptic non-touch technique; make sure you are familiar with it.

☑ Essential equipment

- Suitable personal protective equipment (PPE), in this case, gloves and apron are sufficient
- Bactericidal alcohol hand gel
- A clean tray
- Alcohol wipe (70% alcohol or isopropyl alcohol 70%) (as per local policy)
- Sterile adhesive plaster or hypoallergenic tape
- Sharps bin/receptacle
- *Vacuum system (pre-assembled closed system)
- Appropriate vacuumed specimen tubes
- Disposable tourniquet
- Specimen request forms

*Please note that there are many different pre-assembled vacuum systems available for taking a venous sample of blood. Some vacuum systems are not pre-assembled. Whatever vacuum system you use, it is important to follow the manufacturer's instructions.

☑ Care-setting considerations

If you are carrying out this procedure in a community setting, please ensure that you have a portable sharps box and follow local policy guidelines for the disposal of sharps.

☑ Field-specific considerations

When caring for a patient with a learning disability, it is important to know their level of understanding so that consent for and cooperation with the procedure can be gained. You will need to allow time to explain why you are taking blood and whether the procedure will cause discomfort or pain.

Patients who have mental health problems or those with a learning disability may not understand the relevance of why you need to take blood. They may therefore withhold consent to have their blood taken and you may need to refer to the Mental Capacity Act 2005 and best interest.

☑ What to watch out for and action to take

- Vacutainer system choice: consider – butterfly system should only be used with children or frail, elderly adults. Consider also the gauge of needle used (refer to Appendix 1: Blood Collection Needles).
- The environment: consider – adequate lighting, ventilation, privacy.
- Positioning: consider – operator and patient.
- Choice of vein – involve the patient.
- Consider – venous access devices, skin integrity, surgery, swelling, allergic reactions.
- Please check all packaging before opening: expiry date, packaging undamaged.
- Troubleshoot – methods of vein dilation to improve venous access.
- Follow Moving and Handling policy.

☑ Helpful hints

- Gloves and aprons must be worn if contact with blood/body fluids/excreta is anticipated, or the patient is in isolation.
- Hand hygiene must be performed before touching a patient, before clean/aseptic procedures, after body fluid exposure/risk, after touching a patient and after touching a patient's surroundings.

- Waste should be disposed of in a clinical waste bag if appropriate.
- Sharps should be disposed of following local policy.

Venepuncture: step by step

(1) Introduce yourself to the patient, explain the procedure and gain consent
Fully informed consent may not always be possible if the patient is a child, has mental health problems or has learning disabilities. To alleviate fear and anxiety, every effort should be made to explain the procedure in terms that the patient can understand. In the case of patients who are unable to provide consent because they are unconscious, advice should be sought from your practice educator or another registered nurse

(2) Ask the patient if they have any preferences or experienced any problems during previous venepuncture attempts
Allows the patient to feel involved with the treatment and allows the nurse to assess previous venous history

(3) Check patient identification by asking full name and date of birth. Check information is consistent with request form and identification bracelet if in a hospital setting
To ensure blood is taken from the correct person (NPSA, 2007; RCN, 2010)

(4) Gather the equipment required for venepuncture (see checklist for equipment required)
To ensure you are organised and well prepared for the procedure

(5) Wash hands with bactericidal soap and water before you undertake the procedure and adhere to your local personal protective equipment policy. Check hands for any visibly broken skin, and cover with a waterproof dressing
To minimise the risk of contamination and infection (NHS National Services Scotland, 2012)

6 Take all the equipment to the patient and ensure that patient is in a comfortable position, either sitting on a chair or resting on a bed with arm supported by a pillow
Promotes patient comfort, reduces anxiety and allows good access to veins to perform procedure

7 Apply a tourniquet, at least 5 cm above needle insertion point, making sure it does not obstruct arterial flow
To dilate and increase the prominence of the veins by obstructing the venous return (Dougherty, 2008)

8 Using non-gloved fingers, select the vein carefully by palpation to determine size, depth and condition
Direct skin contact enhances the sense of touch to ensure accurate selection of an appropriate vein and to prevent potential injury to surrounding area

9 Put on gloves
To reduce the risk of contamination

10 Cleanse the patient's skin for 30 seconds using an alcohol wipe (following local policy), in a circular motion from inside to outwards and allow skin to dry. Do not re-palpate or touch the skin
To reduce the risk of infection and contamination

11 Depending on system used, lift needle guard and remove needle sheath carefully and inspect device
To detect any equipment faults (RCN, 2010) and ensure device fully working

12 Apply skin traction a few centimetres below needle insertion point to ensure the vein is anchored
To stabilise the vein

13 Insert the needle at 30° and slightly advance the needle into the vein
To ensure smooth, pain-free needle insertion. To ensure correct position of device

With free hand, insert the vacuumed blood collection bottle (in correct order of draw) onto the device and allow to fill
To ensure accurate volume of blood is drawn and minimise additive contamination from one bottle to another (as manufacturer's guidelines)

 Remove bottle from device and release tourniquet
To prevent blood spillage and to decrease the pressure within vein

 Gently invert the blood bottles according to manufacturer's guidelines
To mix blood with contained additives

 Remove the needle and immediately discard into sharps receptacle
To prevent needle stick injury

 When needle removed apply pressure to puncture site with low-lint swab
To stop blood leakage and prevent complications such as haematoma and bruising

 Assess the puncture site and apply an adhesive plaster or alternative dressing (check allergy status)
To ensure bleeding has stopped

 Before leaving the patient, label the bottles
To ensure the requested blood sample is taken from the correct patient and sent to the laboratory with corresponding patient details

 Discard PPE, any single-use equipment and other used materials as per policy
To prevent cross-infection

 Ensure the patient is comfortable
To check overall well-being post-procedure

 Perform hand hygiene
To minimise risk of infection (NHS National Services Scotland, 2012)

Follow local policy for specimen collection and transportation to laboratory
To ensure timely uplift

Document the procedure in patient's records immediately
Maintains patient safety and accurate records (NMC, 2018)

Source: NHS National Services Scotland (2012); Dougherty (2008); Dougherty and Lister (2015); NPSA (2007); NMC (2018); RCN (2010)

References

Dougherty, L. (2008) 'Obtaining peripheral venous access', in Dougherty, L. and Lamb, J. (eds) *Intravenous Therapy in Nursing Practice*, 2nd edn. Oxford: Blackwell Publishing, pp. 225-70.

Dougherty, L. and Lister, S.E. (eds) (2015) *The Royal Marsden Manual of Clinical Nursing Procedures*, 9th edn. Chichester: Wiley-Blackwell.

Mental Capacity Act (2005) Available at: www.legislation.gov.uk/ukpga/2005/9/pdfs/ukpga_20050009_en.pdf (accessed 10 August 2018).

National Patient Safety Agency (NPSA) (2007) *Standardising Wristbands Improves Patient Safety*. London: NPSA.

NHS National Services Scotland (2012) National Infection Prevention and Control Manual. Available at: www.nipcm.hps.scot.nhs.uk/chapter-1-standard-infection-control-precautions-sicps/#a1069 (accessed 23 January 2019).

Nursing and Midwifery Council (NMC) (2018) The Code: Professional Standards of Practice and Behaviour for Nurses, Midwives and Nursing Associates. London: NMC. Available at: www.nmc.org.uk/globalassets/sitedocuments/nmc-publications/nmc-code.pdf (accessed 16 December 2018).

Royal College of Nursing (RCN) (2010) *Standards for Infusion Therapy*, 3rd edn. London: RCN.

PERIPHERAL IV CANNULATION

WINNIE MCGARRY AND CAROLINE MACCALLUM

☑ Before you start

Remember the common steps for all care delivered to assist patients. This procedure uses the aseptic non-touch technique: make sure you are familiar with it.

☑ Essential equipment

- Suitable personal protective equipment (PPE), in this case gloves and apron are sufficient
- Bactericidal alcohol hand gel
- A clean tray
- Alcohol wipe (70% alcohol or isopropyl alcohol 70%) (as per local policy)
- Low-linting swabs
- Sterile dressing
- Sharps bin/receptacle
- Cannula*
- Disposable tourniquet
- Normal saline to flush cannula (prefilled)

*Ensure correct gauge of cannula is selected.

☑ Care-setting considerations

If you are carrying out this procedure in a community setting, please ensure that you have a portable sharps box and follow local policy guidelines for the disposal of sharps.

- The environment: consider - adequate lighting, ventilation, privacy.
- Positioning: consider - operator and patient.
- Choice of vein - involve the patient.
- If topical local anaesthetic required then this should be applied 30-60 minutes before cannulation attempt (British Medical Association and Royal Pharmaceutical Society, 2014).
- Consider - venous access devices, skin integrity, surgery, swelling, allergic reactions.
- Please check all packaging before opening: expiry date, packaging undamaged.
- Troubleshoot - methods of vein dilation to improve venous access.
- Follow Moving and Handling policy.

☑ Helpful hints

- Gloves and aprons must be worn if contact with blood/body fluids/excreta is anticipated, or the patient is in isolation.
- Hand hygiene must be performed before touching a patient, before clean/aseptic procedures, after body fluid exposure/risk, after touching a patient and after touching a patient's surroundings.
- Waste should be disposed of in a clinical waste bag if appropriate.
- Sharps should be disposed of following local policy.

Peripheral cannulation: step by step

Introduce yourself to the patient, explain the procedure and gain consent

Fully informed consent may not always be possible if the patient is a child, has mental health problems or has learning disabilities. To alleviate fear and anxiety, every effort should be made to explain the procedure in terms that the patient can understand. In the case of patients who are unable to provide consent because they are unconscious, advice should be sought from your practice educator or another registered nurse

2 **Ask the patient if they have any preferences or experienced any problems during previous cannulation experience**
Allows the patient to feel involved with the treatment and allows the nurse to assess previous venous history. If topical local anaesthetic required then this should be applied 30-60 minutes before cannulation attempt (British Medical Association and Royal Pharmaceutical Society, 2014)

3 **Check patient identification by asking full name and date of birth. Check information is consistent with identification bracelet if in a hospital setting**
To ensure peripheral cannula is inserted into the correct person (NPSA, 2007; RCN, 2010)

4 **Gather the equipment required (see checklist for equipment required)**
To ensure you are organised and well prepared for the procedure

5 **Wash hands with bactericidal soap and water before you undertake the procedure and adhere to your local personal protective equipment policy. Check hands for any visibly broken skin, and cover with a waterproof dressing.**
To minimise the risk of contamination and infection (NHS National Services Scotland, 2012)

6 **Take all the equipment to the patient and ensure that the patient is in a comfortable position, either sitting on a chair or resting on a bed with their arm supported by a pillow**
Promotes patient comfort, reduces anxiety and allows good access to veins to perform procedure

7 **Apply a tourniquet, at least 5 cm above cannula insertion point, making sure it does not obstruct arterial flow**
To dilate and increase the prominence of the veins by obstructing the venous return (Dougherty, 2008)

8 **Using non-gloved fingers, select the vein carefully by palpation to determine size, depth and condition**
Direct skin contact enhances the sense of touch to ensure accurate selection of an appropriate vein and to prevent potential injury to surrounding area (Dougherty, 2008; RCN, 2010)

9 Put on gloves
To reduce the risk of contamination

10 Prime the extension set with a syringe of 0.9% sodium chloride (unless taking blood samples immediately after cannulation)
To remove air from the set prior to connection. If taking blood then the sodium chloride will contaminate the sample (Dougherty, 2008)

11 Cleanse the patient's skin for 30 seconds using an alcohol wipe (following local policy). Do not re-palpate or touch the skin
To reduce the risk of infection and contamination

12 Remove needle guard and inspect device
To detect any equipment faults (RCN, 2010) and ensure device fully working

13 Anchor the vein with the non-dominant hand by applying skin traction a few centimetres below needle insertion point
To stabilise the vein and provide counter tension allowing smooth needle entry (Dougherty, 2008)

14 Insert the needle, bevel-up at approximately 30° (depending on vein depth angle may vary) into the skin and slightly advance the needle into the vein
To ensure smooth, pain-free needle insertion (Dougherty, 2008). To ensure correct position of device

15 Wait and observe for flashback of blood in the chamber of the device
To confirm successful vein entry

16 Decrease the angle between the cannula and the skin. Then advance the cannula slightly to ensure entry into the lumen of the vein
To stabilise the device and avoid damage to the vein wall (Dougherty, 2008)

17 Withdraw the needle slightly with the dominant hand and observe for a second flashback of blood along the shaft of the cannula
To ensure correct position of cannula

18 Slowly advance the cannula from the needle into the vein while maintaining skin traction with the non-dominant hand
To stabilise the vein and avoid the risk of vein puncture (Dougherty, 2008)

19 Release the tourniquet
To reduce the pressure within the vein

20 Apply pressure to the vein above the level of the cannula while removing the needle
To avoid spillage of blood

21 Immediately discard needle into sharps receptacle
To prevent needle stick injury

22 If appropriate (depending on device used) attach a primed extension set, needleless injection cap or administration set
To enable flushing of cannula (Dougherty, 2008)

23 While securely holding the device in place, check for blood flashback again then flush the cannula with 0.9% sodium chloride
To stabilise device whilst checking patency (Dougherty, 2008; Goode et al., 1991)

24 Secure with appropriate dressing
To ensure security of device and allow for patient comfort (Dougherty, 2008)

25 Observe the site for signs of swelling or leakage and ask the patient if they are experiencing any discomfort or pain
To ensure device is positioned correctly and secure (Dougherty, 2008)

26 Discard PPE, any single-use equipment and other used materials as per policy
To prevent cross-infection

27 After performing the task, ensure the patient is in a comfortable position, with drinks and call bells available as necessary
Promotes patient comfort and ensures they are well nourished and hydrated

Perform hand hygiene
To minimise risk of infection (NHS National Services Scotland (2012))

Document date, time of insertion, size and site of cannula, number of attempts and any concerns noted in patient's records immediately
Maintains patient safety and accurate records (NMC, 2018)

Source: British Medical Association and Royal Pharmaceutical Society (2014); NHS National Services (2012); Dougherty (2008); Dougherty and Lister (2015); Goode et al. (1991); NMC (2018); NPSA (2007); RCN (2010)

References

British Medical Association and Royal Pharmaceutical Society (2014) *British National Formulary 67*. London: Pharmaceutical Press.

Dougherty, L. (2008) 'Obtaining peripheral vascular access', in Dougherty, L. and Lamb, J. (eds) *Intravenous Therapy in Nursing Practice*, 2nd edn. Oxford: Blackwell Publishing, pp. 225-70.

Dougherty, L. and Lister, S.E. (eds) (2015) *The Royal Marsden Manual of Clinical Nursing Procedures*, 9th edn. Chichester: Wiley-Blackwell.

Goode, C.J., Titler, M., Rakel, B., Ones, D.S., Kleiber, C., Small, S. et al. (1991) 'A meta-analysis of effects of heparin flush and saline flush: Quality and cost implications', *Nursing Research*, *40*(6): 324-30.

National Patient Safety Agency (NPSA) (2007) *Standardising Wristbands Improves Patient Safety*. London: NPSA.

NHS National Services Scotland (2012) National Infection Prevention and Control Manual. Available at: www.nipcm.hps.scot.nhs.uk/chapter-1-standard-infection-control-precautions-sicps/#a1069 (accessed 23 January 2019).

Nursing and Midwifery Council (NMC) (2018) The Code: Professional Standards of Practice and Behaviour for Nurses, Midwives and Nursing Associates. London: NMC. Available at: www.nmc.org.uk/globalassets/sitedocuments/nmc-publications/nmc-code.pdf (accessed 16 December 2018)

Royal College of Nursing (RCN) (2010) *Standards for Infusion Therapy*, 3rd edn. London: RCN.

INTRAVENOUS FLUIDS

MEGHAN BATESON AND LIZANNE HAMILTON-SMITH

Introduction

Intravenous (IV) fluids are commonly prescribed to hospitalised patients. As IV fluids are drugs their administration must be carefully managed (see Appendix 2: Fluid Status Assessment).

☑ **Care-setting considerations**

Calculating the rate

> **Using a volumetric pump:** The rate of an IV fluid infusion being administered by pump should be prescribed as millilitres per hour. Follow local policy in the use of volumetric pumps by student nurses. Always seek training on the pump used in your clinical area prior to using the device.

> **Using a gravity infusion:** Gravity infusions are used without a pump and the rate is calculated as drop rate or drops per minute. The drop rate is equal to how many drops you watch enter the drip chamber of the administration set every minute. To calculate the drop rate you need to know the drop factor of the administration set. This can be found on the packaging of the administration set.

The calculation for the drop rate of a gravity infusion is:

$$\text{Number of drops per minute} = \frac{\text{Volume of infusion fluid} \times \text{Drop factor}}{\text{Duration of infusion in minutes}}$$

Example:

A patient is prescribed 500 ml sodium chloride (NaCl) 0.9% to be administered over 4 hours. How many drops per minute should the gravity infusion be set to?

Volume = 500 ml

Duration = 4 hours = $4 \times 60 = 240$ minutes

Drop factor = 20 gtt

$$\frac{500 \times 20}{240} = 42 \text{ drops per minute}$$

☑ Essential equipment

- Hand hygiene gel
- Non-sterile gloves
- Volumetric pump if required
- IV fluid administration set (select the correct administration set for the method of administration, e.g. a volumetric pump will require a different administration set from a gravity infusion)
- Alcohol or 2% chlorhexidine swab ×2 (one for cleaning the port on the infusion bag and one for cleaning the hub of the IV access device)
- Equipment for flushing IV cannula
- Infusion bag
- Drip stand

☑ What to watch out for and action to take

- The environment: consider - adequate lighting, ventilation, privacy.
- Positioning: consider - operator and patient.
- Please check all packaging before opening: expiry date, packaging undamaged.
- Follow Moving and Handling policy.
- The colour of the skin, lips and nail beds for signs of cyanosis.
- The patient's positioning and how they are moving.
- Their neurological condition - are they alert and responsive?
- Any signs of pain or discomfort.
- The patient's or relatives' views - for example, saying their condition is 'not quite right' or they 'don't feel well'.

- Colloids carry an anaphylaxis risk and some products are not suitable for vegetarians, vegans and people of religions who do not consume certain animal products.
- Hand hygiene must be performed before touching a patient, before clean/aseptic procedures, after body fluid exposure/risk, after touching a patient and after touching a patient's surroundings.
- Waste should be disposed of in a clinical waste bag if appropriate.
- Particular things to be aware of for IV fluid administration are:
  - What is the IV fluid plan for this patient?
  - What happens after this bag finishes? Are any further infusions prescribed?
  - When is the patient next due an assessment of their fluid status?
  - What is the prescribed volume of the fluid to be infused (e.g. 500 ml)?
  - What rate is the fluid to be infused at?
  - Check site of infusion, e.g. peripheral venous cannula (see Peripheral IV Cannualtion chapter for care and what to look out for).
  - If new cannula is required it must be replaced.
  - Check prescription and bag for any included additives, e.g. potassium.
  - Check that the outer packaging of infusion bag is intact without any punctures, leakage or crusting.
  - Check that the fluid in the bag is clear and free from any particles, cloudiness or discolouration.

IV Fluids: step by Step

Introduce yourself to the patient, explain the procedure and gain consent

Fully informed consent may not always be possible if the patient is a child, has mental health problems or has learning disabilities. To alleviate fear and anxiety, every effort should be made to explain the procedure in terms that the patient can understand. In the case of patients who are unable to provide consent because they are unconscious, advice should be sought from your practice educator or another registered nurse

(2) Check patient identification by asking full name and date of birth. Check information is consistent with identification bracelet if in a hospital setting
To ensure peripheral cannula is inserted into the correct person (NPSA, 2007; RCN, 2010)

(3) Gather the equipment required (see checklist for equipment required)
To ensure you are organised and well prepared for the procedure

(4) Wash hands with bactericidal soap and water before you undertake the procedure and adhere to your local personal protective equipment policy. Check hands for any visibly broken skin, and cover with a waterproof dressing
To minimise the risk of contamination and infection (NHS National Services Scotland, 2012)

(5) Take all the equipment to the patient and ensure that the patient is in a comfortable position, either sitting on a chair or resting on a bed with their arm supported by a pillow
Promotes patient comfort, reduces anxiety and allows good access to veins to perform procedure

(6) Check the prescription
The general principles of medication administration are the same for administration of IV fluids - please review the Medicines administration chapter

(7) Prime the administration set by opening the administration set packaging. Clamp off roller clamp
To prime the equipment for infusion

(8) Remove infusion bag from packaging
To enable connection to the administration set

(9) Remove protective cap from insertion port on infusion bag
To enable connection of the infusion solution to the administration set

10 **Clean infusion port with alcohol swab for 30 seconds**
To reduce the risk of infection and contamination

11 **Remove cap from spike on administration set**
To enable connection to the infusion solution

12 **Using a half screwing motion insert the spike into the port in the infusion bag**
To ensure effective connection

13 **Hang spiked bag on drip stand**
To enable effective priming of the solution to be administered

14 **Fill the drip chamber (the cylinder below the spike) by squeezing and releasing the chamber until the fluid reaches approximately half way up the chamber**
To enable effective priming of the administration set

15 **Slowly unclamp the roller clamp and allow the fluid to prime the administration set to the point at which it would attach to the patient**
To enable effective priming of the solution to be administered within the administration set

16 **If there are small bubbles of air, flick the tubing with your finger and allow the bubbles to rise up to the end of the administration set and then allow these to flush out into a clean receptacle**
To minimise risk of infusing air and to promote patient safety

17 **Clamp off the roller clamp**
To prevent leakage prior to administration

18 **Connection to the patient**
The role of the student nurse in connecting IV fluids is subject to local and regional policy. Please check and ensure that you adhere to the policy in your university and clinical placement areas

19 **Clean the hub of the IV cannula or needle free access with an alcohol swab**
To minimise infection

(20) **Flush IV cannula as per local policy**
To maintain the patency of the device

(21) **Before connecting to patient, unclamp roller clamp briefly to ensure fluid right to tip of the administration set (no air bubble in line)**
To ensure patency of the tube

(22) **Connect administration set to IV cannula**
To commence the infusion

(23) **The roller clamp can now be open**
To check the infusion is now flowing

(24) **Calculating the drip rate**
To ensure the patient receives the correct dose of fluids (see considerations above)

(25) **Documentation**
Once the IV infusion has started, the documentation should be completed as per local policy. This usually includes:

- date/time of start
- IV pump chart documentation if required
- batch number of infusion bag
- expiry date
- signed by two registered nurses (check local policy)

To maintain patient safety and accurate record keeping

(26) **Monitoring the infusion: follow guidance in the Peripheral IV Cannulation chapter about site monitoring and maintenance rate of infusion**

- **Volumetric pump:** Pump chart documentation should be completed hourly and updated with any rate or bag changes to reflect: time, rate, volume to be infused, volume already infused, and signature of nurse
- **Gravity infusion:** Regularly re-count drops per minute to ensure that set rate is being maintained. The rate can inadvertently change due to patient positioning

To maintain patient safety and identify any changes to insertion site

End of the infusion bag - disconnection
The role of the student nurse in disconnecting IV fluids is subject to local and regional policy. Please ensure that you adhere to the policy in your university and clinical placement areas

If permitted to disconnect:

 Gather: non-sterile gloves for handling peripheral venous cannula, sterile bung, equipment of IV flush as per local policy
To reduce the chance of infection and maintain patient and nurse safety

 Close roller clamp
To stop the flow of the infusion

 Disconnect IV tubing and connect sterile bung if no needle free access device in use
To maintain a closed system

 Flush IV cannula as per local policy
To maintain the patency of the cannula

 Document volume infused on input/output chart as per local policy (see Appendix 3: Intake/Output Charts)
To maintain patient safety and identify any changes to insertion site

Source: NICE (2013)

References

National Institute for Health and Care Excellence (NICE) (2013) *Intravenous Fluid Therapy in Adults in Hospital*. Clinical Guideline 174. London: NICE.
National Patient Safety Agency (NPSA) (2007) *Standardising Wristbands Improves Patient Safety*. London: NPSA.

NHS National Services Scotland (2012) National Infection Prevention and Control Manual. Available at: www.nipcm.hps.scot.nhs.uk/chapter-1-standard-infection-control-precautions-sicps/#a1069 (accessed 23 January 2019).

Royal College of Nursing (RCN) (2010) *Standards for Infusion Therapy*, 3rd edn. London: RCN.

BLOOD TRANSFUSION

SALLY RICHARDSON AND KAREN ELLIOTT

A blood transfusion is the administration of whole blood or a blood component directly into a vein. There are risks associated with blood transfusion. Bolton-Maggs et al. (2015) identify the biggest risks as the pre-transfusion checks and correct patient identification. The actual risk posed by the transfusion can be minimised by reducing the unnecessary use of blood, alongside the use of hospital policy and procedures throughout.

☑ Before you start

- Ensure that suitably trained staff are available throughout the transfusion - this must be appropriately IV trained health care practitioners (HCPs). Only authorised trained, competent and designated staff can collect blood from the blood designated fridges (Blood Safety and Quality Regulations standards SI 2005 No. 50 as amended).
- Be aware that only one unit of blood should be collected at a time unless directed otherwise - this would be associated with emergency situations.
- Ensure the patient's baseline observations have been completed, documented and assessed as acceptable to start transfusion.

☑ Essential equipment

- Blood-giving set with a double chamber and a standard 170-200 micron filter
- IV infusion drip stand

Consider if the following equipment is required:

- infusion pump – might be required depending on local policy or for high risk patients
- rapid infusion devices – if large transfusions are to be given, usually in an emergency
- blood warmer – not generally recommended but consider for large volume transfusions or high risk patients.

All of the above equipment must be used in line with local policy and in accordance with the manufacturer's instructions/guidelines.

☑ Care-setting considerations

- Ensure the transfusion is necessary and the patient has consented.
- Ensure and check all documentation is in place before you start.
- Consider the patient's blood group and ensure this is documented with crossmatch reference.
- Time-management: plan timings – once blood is collected from the fridge transfusion should be started without delay.
- Know and adhere to local policy and guidelines.

☑ What to watch out for and action to take

- Allergic reactions
- Circulatory overload
- Haemolytic reaction
- Haemolytic febrile reaction
- Drop in blood pressure – hypotension
- Increased pulse rate – tachycardia
- Drop in urine output
- Pain at cannula site
- Back or loin pain
- Changes to breathing
- Rash
- Restlessness or signs of distress
- Raise in temperature >1.5 °C

ACTION: Any signs above = STOP INFUSION

☑ **Helpful hints**

- Refer to and pre-read relevant local policy.
- PPE – gloves should be used when there is risk of contact with the blood product.
- Hand hygiene should be hand-washing with soap and water initially and the use of a non-touch technique.
- If in doubt at any point – stop the infusion.

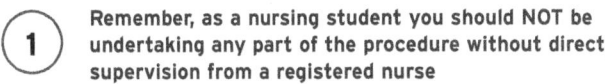

Blood transfusion: step by step

1 **Remember, as a nursing student you should NOT be undertaking any part of the procedure without direct supervision from a registered nurse**
To ensure patient safety and to guide and support your own learning

2 **Introduce yourself to the patient and confirm their identity, ensuring an ID bracelet is in place: explain the procedure and ensure their understanding of the blood transfusion**
Informed consent implies that the patient should have insight into the associated risks, benefits, consequences and any alternatives to a blood transfusion. This assists in the delivery of the procedure as the patient has an understanding of and is compliant with care, hopefully reducing any anxieties.

Not all patients will consent due to age, capacity, clinical condition, religious beliefs, and ethical concerns; in these situations seek help and advice from a qualified HCP.

3 **Ensure the blood transfusion is documented within the patient's notes and prescribed by an authorised HCP. Pre-transfusion documentation should include:**

- **the clinical indication for the transfusion**
- **patient's body weight**
- **date of clinical decision to transfuse and date of planned transfusion**

- **blood components to be transfused, and volume, dose, rate/duration of the transfusion**
- **patient consent**
- **the ID of person making the decision to transfuse/ or authorising the transfusion**

(Robinson et al., 2017)

To ensure patient safety and ensure an appropriate documentation trail is evident

(4) **Measure, record and document an initial baseline observation, to be no more than 60 minutes before the transfusion begins**
To ensure patient safety and comfort for the blood transfusion to be administered

(5) **Check the patient has appropriate and working IV access for the transfusion to be delivered. This could be a peripherally inserted central catheter (PICC), or central venous catheter (CVC)**
To ensure patient safety and comfort for the blood transfusion to be administered. Any IV access must be checked in line with local policy and assessment tools such as Visual Infusion Phlebitis (VIP) score (INS, 2011)

(6) **Arrange with authorised staff for one blood unit collection from the blood fridge. Correct patient documentation must be taken to allow for the completion of the blood bank register. This will include:**

- **the patient's hospital number**
- **the unique number of the red blood cells**
- **the date and time of collection**
- **the name of the person collecting the unit and signature**

To ensure the correct guidelines and local policies are adhered to, thus ensuring patient safety. The appropriate documentation must be completed at the time of blood collection to maintain the blood bank register

(7) **Once documentation is completed, the blood unit should be transferred within approximately 30 minutes to the clinical area. Transfer within an appropriate cool box should be considered if longer than 30 minutes is needed to complete this process**

To reduce the risk of deterioration, warming and potential for bacterial growth in the blood product (Norfolk, 2013), thus ensuring patient safety

 Check the prescription against the unit of blood. This should include: date, volume, rate, signature, and any special requirements

The calculation of the required infusion drip rate should be made using the correct formula:

$$\frac{\text{Volume}}{\text{Time}} \times \frac{\text{Drops per ml}}{60} = \text{Drops per minute}$$

Any medication should be prescribed by an authorised HCP and should be clearly signed.

Any queries at this stage should be checked with the prescriber.

All checks should usually be carried out with two checkers, one of whom should be a registered HCP, or in line with local policy

 Gather equipment for the procedure, including:

- **IV infusion stand**
- **sterile blood-giving set**
- **gloves**
- **alcohol gel**

To ensure the smooth process of preparing and setting up the transfusion. This avoids leaving the patient and ensures timely administration of the blood transfusion

 Check patient identification again via ID bracelet and verbally, cross-referencing with the documentation, prescription and blood labelling (NPSA, 2006). In addition, the blood expiry date must be checked Note: Some areas might also use technology such as bar code scanning within this process; follow local policy To ensure the correct guidelines and local policies are adhered to, ensuring patient safety

The appropriate documentation must be completed prior to the time of administration in line with the medication administration standards

(11) **Wash hands with soap and water and apply non-sterile gloves**
Hang the blood bag/unit on the IV infusion stand
To prevent cross contamination

(12) **Check the giving set expiry date, open it using a non-touch technique, then turn the roller clamp to the off/closed position (fully down)**
To ensure sterility and prevent air embolus

(13) **Using a non-touch technique, remove the protective spike cover from the giving set and insert the sterile spike into the hanging blood bag**
To connect the blood bag and giving set

(14) **Allow blood to drip into the chamber, gently squeezing as required to the fill line**
To prevent air embolus

(15) **Open the roller clamp to allow the blood to slowly drip and prime the giving set line, checking for any air or bubbles as this is done**
To prime the line and prevent air embolus

(16) **Close the clamp when the line is fully primed and no air is visible**
To prevent blood leakage from the giving set

(17) **The line is now ready to be attached to the patient. Connect the giving set to the cannula/IV device using a non-touch technique. This must be done by a trained and registered HCP**

Open the roller clamp and set the flow rate at the correct calculated drip rate
To ensure the correct guidelines and local policies are adhered to, thus ensuring patient safety.

Ensure the patient is resting comfortably and that their arm is well supported to prevent interruption to the transfusion flow rate

(18) Documentation must be completed within the prescription and the start time of the blood transfusion noted
The prescription chart should be completed and signed by the HCPs involved; documentation is also recorded within the patient notes

(19) Fifteen minutes after the transfusion start time the first set of observations must be taken, documented and compared with the baseline observations

If stable then continue to monitor the patient for any adverse reactions for the remainder of the transfusion unless the patient's clinical condition warrants further observations being repeated
Observations should be undertaken in accordance with local policy and dependent on the patient's condition during the transfusion

(20) On completion of the blood transfusion, close the roller clamp and, whilst still wearing gloves, disconnect the blood bag using a non-touch technique. This should be disposed of in clinical waste in accordance with local policy
To ensure the correct guidelines and local policies are adhered to, ensuring both staff and patient safety

(21) A final set of observations should be recorded and documented in the notes. Should the patient require an additional blood transfusion this should now be connected and started. Transfusion documentation must be completed and the blood tag returned to the blood bank (BSQR, 2005)
To ensure the correct guidelines, local and national policies are adhered to, ensuring both staff and patient safety

References

Bolton-Maggs, P.H.B. and Cohen, H. (2013) 'Serious Hazards of Transfusion (SHOT) haemovigilance and progress is improving transfusion safety', *British Journal of Haematology*, *163* (3): 303-14.

Infusion Nurses Society (INS) (2011) 'Infusion nursing standards of practice', *Journal of Infusion Nursing*, *34*(1 supplement).

National Patient Safety Agency (NSPA) (2006) *Safer Practice Notice 14: Right Patient, Right Blood.* Available at: https://webarchive.national archives.gov.uk/20100311015613/http://www.nrls.npsa.nhs.uk/ resources/search-by-audience/midwife/?entryid45=59805&cid=8 98358&p=1 (accessed 17 December 2018).

Norfolk, D. (2013) *Handbook of Transfusion Medicine: Blood Transfusion Services of the United Kingdom*, 5th edn. Norwich: TSO.

Nursing and Midwifery Council (NMC) (2015) Standards for Medicine Management. London: NMC.

Robinson, S,. Harris, A., Atkinson, S. et al. (2017) 'The administration of blood components: A British society for haematology guideline', *Transfusion Medicine*, *28*(1): 3-21.

The Blood Safety and Quality Regulations (BSQR) (2005) Available at: www. legislation.gov.uk/uksi/2005/50/made (accessed 18 September 2018).

CENTRAL VENOUS ACCESS DEVICES

KAMALPREET KAUR DHINDSA

A central venous catheter (CVC) is a catheter with a tip that lies within the proximal third of the superior vena cava, the right atrium, or the inferior vena cava. Catheters can be inserted through a peripheral vein or a proximal central vein, most commonly the internal jugular, subclavian or a femoral vein (Smith and Nolan, 2013).

☑ **Before you start**

- Insertion is performed by a competent HCP with assistance.
- Informed consent should be obtained before beginning the procedure.
- Gather all the necessary equipment before insertion.
- Choice of device is made based on the indications and duration the catheter is needed for.

Table 2 Types of CVC and indications for insertion

Type of line	Site of insertion	Expected duration	Indications
Non-tunnelled	Internal jugular vein, subclavian vein, axillary vein, femoral vein	Short term (several days to 3-4 weeks)	Difficult IV access; infusion of irritant drugs, vasopressors, inotropes; short term total parenteral nutrition (TPN). Mainly inserted in critical care units

(Continued)

Table 2 (Continued)

Type of line	Site of insertion	Expected duration	Indications
PICC (Peripherally inserted central catheters)	Basilic vein, cephalic vein, brachial vein	Weeks to months	Difficult intravenous access; blood sampling; medium term drug administration (for example, antibiotics); administration of irritant drugs (such as chemotherapy); TPN
Tunnelled (e.g. Hickman, Groshong)	Internal jugular vein, subclavian vein	Long term (months to years)	Long term administration of irritant drugs (chemotherapy)
Implantable ports	Internal jugular vein, subclavian vein	Long term (months to years)	Long term intermittent access, for example, regular hospital admissions with poor intravenous access, administration of irritant drugs (chemotherapy)

☑ **Potential contraindications to CVC insertion (Smith and Nolan, 2013)**

- Coagulopathy
- Thrombocytopenia
- Ipsilateral haemothorax or pneumothorax
- Vessel thrombosis, stenosis or disruption
- Infection overlying insertion site

Source: Smith and Nolan (2013)

☑ Essential equipment

- Sterile pack containing sterile gown and drapes
- Sterile gloves
- Alcohol hand scrub
- Alcohol skin cleaning preparations as 2% chlorhexidine in 70% alcohol
- 5 ml, 10 ml syringes
- Needleless injection cap
- Introducer
- CVC catheter and insertion kit
- Transparent dressing
- Sutures/securing device
- 21G, 23G, 25G needles
- Ultrasound machine, gel and probe cover
- 0.9% sodium chloride
- 1% lidocaine

☑ Care-setting considerations

Central venous access devices (CVADs) are inserted after careful consideration of the patient's condition and need for a device. CVADs are inserted in specialist areas by trained doctors and nurses. Check local policies when looking after patients with a CVAD.

☑ What to watch out for and action to take

- Observe for signs of infection. If suspected, swab the site and start antibiotics. If the patient shows signs of systemic infection or rigors when flushing the line, take blood cultures from all lumens. Remove the catheter and send the tip for microbiology. Consider sepsis protocol.
- Occlusion is prevented by correct use, technique and frequency of flush. A persistent withdrawal occlusion – when injection is possible, but aspiration is not possible – may be resolved using push lock protocol by bolus or infusion. Only 10 ml or larger syringes should be used. In case of total occlusion, urokinase can be instilled using the three-way tap method. Always check trust policy before making any decisions
- Thrombosis: ultrasound is undertaken to ascertain the size and location of the thrombus and anticoagulant therapy is commenced. The catheter should only be removed after 72 hours of commencing anticoagulant therapy.
- Infiltration and extravasation: stop the infusion and inform a doctor.

- Regularly inspect site for any signs of infection or other complications.
- Use aseptic technique; clean hubs with 2% chlorhexidine in 70% alcohol prior to use.
- Needle free injection caps should be changed weekly or as the policy dictates.
- Dressing should be changed weekly unless the site is bleeding or oozing. Semi-permeable transparent dressing is the first choice. Antimicrobial dressings such as bio patch can be used in patients with high infection risk or in line with hospital policy.
- Maintaining patency: use of a 10 ml syringe or larger is recommended when using CVADs. Flush the catheter using push-pause method. Maintain pressure on the plunger whilst disconnecting the syringe and do not clamp the catheter until the syringe has been disconnected. This must be undertaken by a suitably qualified HCP.
- Blood sampling: must be done using vacuum adopter system. Use needleless injection cap to maintain a closed system. Flush with at least 20 ml sodium chloride (NaCl) after blood sampling.
- Administration sets should be labelled. Change sets immediately following administration of blood and blood products, after 24 hours following TPN and every 96 hours if continuous fluids are administered.

Source: Frimpong et al. (2015); GOSH (2015); NICE (2017); Scales (2013)

Central venous access devices: step by step

(1) **Explain procedure to the patient and obtain informed consent where possible**
The NMC code of conduct requires the nurse to obtain informed consent. May improve patient compliance and cooperation in conscious patients

(2) **Gather all the required equipment, including a CVAD pack**
Use of CVAD pack ensures all equipment is compatible to reduce delays and improve safety

(3) **Connect the patient to bedside ECG monitoring**
To detect dysrhythmias associated with CVAD insertion

4 **Position the patient supine, and head down (if clinically tolerated and appropriate)**
Reduces the risk of air embolism during insertion

5 **The person performing the procedure performs a surgical scrub and dons sterile gown and gloves**
Barrier precautions to reduce infection risk

6 **The person assisting opens the packets and passes equipment to the operator using ANTT and without contaminating the sterile field**
To prevent contamination of sterile products and sterile field

7 **The person performing the procedure primes the CVAD with 0.9% sodium chloride**
Prevents air embolism

8 **Skin around the insertion site is prepared using 2% chlorhexidine in 70% alcohol**
To reduce the risk of infection

9 **Fenestrated drape is positioned over the intended insertion site to create a sterile field**
Reduces the risk of infection

10 **The skin around the insertion site is infiltrated with 1% lidocaine solution**
To reduce pain and sensation during insertion

11 **The assistant applies ultrasound gel to the head of the probe. Then a sterile ultrasound probe cover is applied**
To improve conductivity and maintain sterility

12 **Using ultrasound, a needle mounted onto a syringe is inserted into the vein. Once blood is freely aspirated, the syringe is removed from the needle**
Use of CVAD pack ensures all equipment is compatible, to reduce delays and improve safety. Blood flow ensures correct placement of the catheter in the vein

13 **Carefully maintaining the needle position within the vein, a J-wire is advanced through the barrel of the syringe and the wire is threaded into the vein. The ECG monitor should be observed for any changes of the rhythm**
J-wire has a rounded flexible tip that reduces the risk of vein wall puncture. ECG changes indicate the guidewire is in the heart

14 If the wire threads easily into the vein, the needle and syringe are removed
Care is taken not to remove the wire at the same time

15 The needle is removed and a dilator is advanced over the guide wire up to the puncture site
To aid the advancement of the catheter through the skin

16 A small incision is made in the skin at the puncture site. The dilator is then advanced using a gentle corkscrew motion to dilate the soft tissue
To aid the advancement of the catheter through the skin

17 The central lumen of the CVAD is passed over the guidewire and is carefully advanced through the skin until the wire appears at the end of the catheter. Holding on to the guidewire, the catheter is carefully advanced into the vein
Care must be taken to avoid the guidewire from accidentally being advanced into the vein

18 The guidewire is withdrawn once the catheter is correctly positioned. The end of the catheter must be occluded
Occlusion prevents air embolism

19 Each lumen of the CVAD is aspirated and flushed with 0.9% sodium chloride (NaCl). The insertion site is cleaned with 2% chlorhexidine and 70% alcohol and allowed to dry
Aspiration ensures each lumen is correctly positioned within the vein. Cleaning reduces the growth of microflora

20 The CVAD must be secured using statlock or sutures
Prevents dislodgement

21 The CVAD is dressed with a transparent moisture-permeable dressing
To protect the insertion site and prevent moisture build up

22 The patient should be repositioned comfortably and the CVAD tip should be confirmed on X-ray prior to use
To ensure the catheter tip is in the right position

(23) **Insertion date, insertion site, type of CVAD should be recorded in the patient's medical records**
To ensure correct documentation

Source: Scales (2010)

CVAD removal

- Remove CVAD as soon as it is no longer needed.
- Nurses can remove PICCs but not cuffed CVC.
- Skin tunnelled catheters can be removed using surgical techniques by nurses and doctors.
- Implantable ports are generally removed by surgeons or anaesthetists or specially trained nurses.
- FBCs and coagulation screens are checked prior to removal.

Source: GOSH (2015); NICE (2017)

References

Frimpong, A., Caruioa, J. and Octavo, G. (2015) 'Promoting safe IV management in practice using H.A.N.D.S.', *British Journal of Nursing*, 24(2): S18, S20-3.

Great Ormond Street Hospital for Children (GOSH) (2015) *Central Venous Access Devices (long term)*. Available at: www.gosh.nhs.uk/health-professionals/clinical-guidelines/central-venous-access-devices-long-term (accessed 10 August 2018).

National Institute for Health and Care Excellence (NICE) (2017) *Central Venous Access Devices: Policy for Insertion and Care in Hospital*. Available at: www.nice.org.uk/guidance/mtg34/resources/policy-for-the-insertion-and-care-of-central-venous-access-devices-cvad-in-hospital-royal-marsden-nhs-ft-pdf-4481503169 (accessed 10 August 2018).

Scales, K. (2010) 'Central venous access devices: Part 1 - Devices for acute care', *British Journal of Nursing*, 19(2): 88-92.

Scales, K. (2013) 'Central venous access devices: Part 2 - For intermediate and long term use', *British Journal of Nursing*, 19(Suppl.1): S20-5.

Smith, N.R. and Nolan, P.J. (2013) 'Central venous catheters - Clinical review', *British Medical Journal, 347*: f6570.

ECG

MEGHAN BATESON AND LIZANNE HAMILTON-SMITH

Introduction

Electrocardiograms (ECG) are commonly used to record the electrical activity in the heart. There are two main ways they are used:

12 lead ECG
- Provides 12 different views of the heart's electrical activity using ten leads.
- Printed on ECG paper - graph paper with small squares within larger ones (see Figure 1). The ECG paper moves through the ECG machine at 25 mm per second which allows measurement of size and duration of the ECG waveform.

Continuous cardiac monitoring
- Provides uninterrupted monitoring of a patient's heart usually with either three or five leads.
- Used for patients who are at risk of deterioration, e.g. in intensive care.
- Can produce a rhythm strip printed on ECG paper providing one view of the heart rhythm.

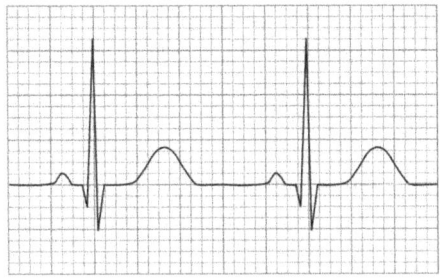

Figure 1 ECG paper

Source: Madhero88 https://commons.wikimedia.org/wiki/File:ECGbasic.svg

☑ **Before you start**

A normal ECG waveform consists of several sections which reflect the journey of a nerve impulse through the heart (see Figure 2). In order to recognise abnormal heart rhythms you must be able to identify and interpret the components of a normal ECG waveform. Please see Appendix 4, ECG Interpretation, for more detail.

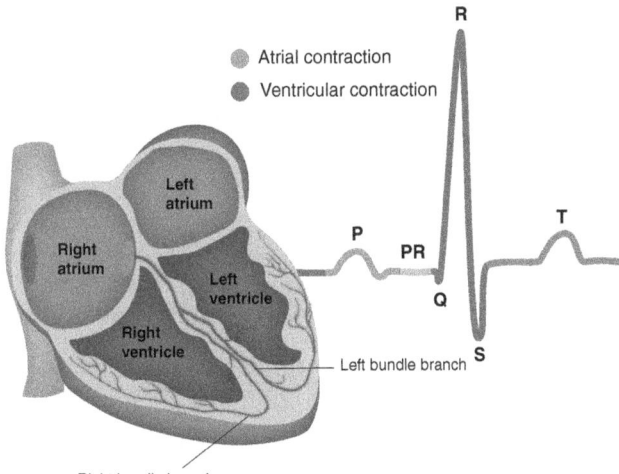

Figure 2 ECG waveform

Source: Boore et al. (2016). Illustrated by Shaun Mercier, © SAGE Publications

- **Offer a chaperone:** ECG monitoring requires exposure of the chest for the application of electrodes.
- **Skin preparation:** Skin must be clean, dry and hair free. Occasionally alcohol wipes to cleanse skin or razor to remove hair are required.
- **Patient position:** For 12 lead ECG the patient should lie supine or at a 45 degree angle, but they can sit higher up if necessary. For continuous cardiac monitoring patients can move around. Monitor for interference or poor trace.
- **Interference:** Interference can result in an inaccurate or unclear ECG. Common sources of interference are the patient speaking or coughing and poor connection between the ECG leads and the electrodes .
- **Poor trace:** Check electrodes have good adherence to the skin and that the patient's condition has not deteriorated. A completely flat line usually indicates a misplaced electrode.

☑ **Essential equipment**

- **Training:** Ensure you have had training on the use of the machine and follow the manufacturer's instructions at all times.
- **Machine:** Check the ECG machine (for 12 lead ECG measurement) or cardiac monitor (for 3 or 5 lead ECGs) is clean, charged or connected to a power supply.
- **Leads:** Check the ECG leads attached to the machine are clean and free from cracks. If any cracks or exposed wires are noted, the machine must be reported to medical physics for repair and another machine located.
- **Electrodes:**
  - 12 lead ECG: Check that you have at least 10 ECG electrodes (the self-adhesive pads used to attach the ECG leads to the patient) which are suitable for use with the ECG machine.
  - 3 or 5 lead ECG: Check that you have 3 or 5 self-adhesive ECG electrodes which are compliant with the cardiac monitor being used.
  - *If the patient has an allergy to the electrodes (evidenced by inflamed or broken skin) use hypoallergenic electrodes.*
- ECG paper: Check the ECG machine is loaded with ECG paper.

- Patient identifier: Ensure the patient's details are either electronically inputted or the patient label attached to the ECG paper and filed correctly to maintain accurate records.

ECG measurement: step by step

1 **The first step of any procedure is to introduce yourself to the patient, explain the procedure and gain their consent**
Fully informed consent may not always be possible if the patient is a child, has mental health problems or has learning disabilities, but even in these circumstances, every effort should be made to explain the procedure in terms that the patient can understand. This is not only respectful of their individual human rights, but also helps to ensure that they will be more accepting of the treatment and that their anxieties are reduced. In the case of patients who are unable to provide consent because they are unconscious, advice should be sought from senior nursing staff and local policies adhered to

2 **Gather the equipment required. Ensure this is clean and in working order**
Promotes patient safety and infection control and reduces the chance of inaccurate readings

3 **Clear sufficient space within the environment, for example around the bed space**
Enables clear access to the patient and safer use of the necessary equipment

4 **Wash your hands with soap and water before you undertake clinical measurements. Apron and gloves should only be worn if appropriate. Consider the individual patient situation and the risk presented**
Promotes patient safety and reduces the risk of infection

5 **Patients should be in a private, comfortable and appropriate position and surroundings**
Maintains patient privacy, dignity and comfort and may help to reduce anxiety

6   **Switch on ECG machine and enter any required information**
Promotes patient safety and prepares the equipment for use

12 lead ECG measurement

Follow preparatory steps 1 to 6 above.

7   **Apply ECG electrodes**

- **There are 10 electrodes placed for a 12 lead ECG. The correct lead must be attached to its allocated anatomical position otherwise the ECG recording will be inaccurate**
- **There are four limb leads (one for each arm and leg) and six chest leads (labelled V1-V6) (see Figure 3)**

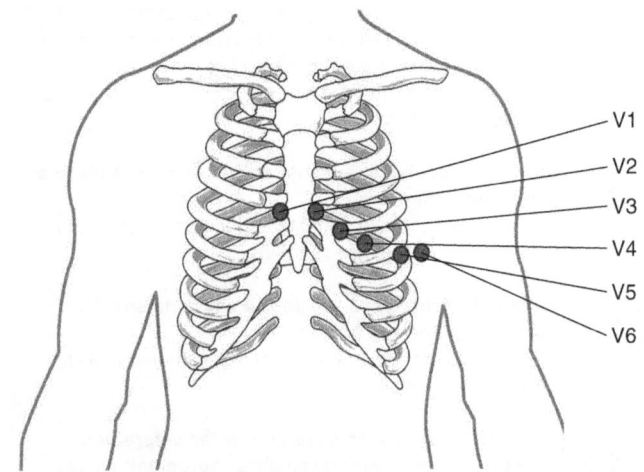

Figure 3   Placement of leads

Source: OpenStax College, Wikipedia Commons (CC BY 3.0)

- **Place the chest leads in the following order:**

    - **V1: 4th intercostal space, right sternal edge. To locate the 4th intercostal space gently move**

two fingers down the patient's sternum until you feel a lump. This is known as the angle of Louis. Move your fingers to the right and feel a gap between the ribs. This is the 2nd intercostal space. From the 2nd intercostal space slide your fingers across the third and fourth ribs and into the 4th intercostal space. Place an electrode for V1 here
  - o V2: 4th intercostal space, left sternal edge. To locate, repeat process above
  - o V4: Midclavicular line (in line with the middle of the left clavicle), 5th intercostal space
  - o V3: Midway between V2 and V4
  - o V5: Anterior axilliary line, 5th intercostal space, on the same horizontal line as V4
  - o V6: Midaxilliary line (middle of left axilla), 5th intercostal space, on the same horizontal line as V4 and V5

- **Place leads V3-V6 under the left breast of female patients.** This may require you to gain consent from the patient for the left breast to be gently lifted (ideally by the patient themselves) to allow accurate lead placement
- **When placing all four limb leads remember that they should be an equal distance away from the heart.** One electrode is usually placed on each wrist and ankle but anywhere up each limb is acceptable so long as the distance to each electrode is roughly equal
- **Ensure electrodes are applied to intact hair free skin** To enable accurate recording to be undertaken

Recording the ECG

- **Once a clear ECG trace is obtained ask the patient to remain still and silent for a moment.** Press record and the ECG machine will print a copy of the 12 lead ECG
- **Ensure patient details (minimum of name, date of birth and patient number) are on the ECG print out**
- **If the patient is experiencing chest pain during the ECG recording, make note of that on the ECG.** If the patient is experiencing new chest pain immediately seek senior nursing and medical assistance

To enable accurate documentation of the recording and to respond immediately to the needs of the patient

(9) **Disconnect the ECG leads from the electrodes and gently remove the electrodes from the skin. Offer cleanser to remove any remaining residue. Inspect the skin to ensure it is intact**
To maintain dignity and to promote patient comfort

(10) **After performing the clinical measurement, ensure the patient is in a comfortable position, with drinks and a call bell available as necessary**
Ensures patient comfort

(11) **Report the ECG to the nursing and medical team for review and interpretation. Ensure ECG filed correctly following interpretation**
Maintains patient safety and accurate records

3 or 5 lead ECG measurement

Follow preparatory steps 1 to 6 above.

(7) **Apply ECG electrodes**

- **For 3 lead ECG monitoring:**
  - o **Red lead: connect to electrode placed under the right clavicle near the right shoulder**
  - o **Yellow lead: connect to electrode under the left clavicle near the left shoulder**
  - o **Green lead: connect to electrode on the left lower edge of the rib cage in the midaxilliary line**

- **For 5 lead ECG monitoring place the leads as per 3 lead monitoring above and add in two additional electrodes:**

- o **White lead: connect to electrode on the 4th intercostal space at the left sternal border – see above in 12 lead ECG placement for how to locate the 4th intercostal space**
- o **Black lead: connect to electrode placed on the lower edge of the right rib cage in the mid axilliary line** To enable an accurate recording to be undertaken

(8) **Confirm clear ECG trace**
To enable accurate documentation and to maintain patient safety

(9) **After performing the clinical measurement, ensure the patient is in a comfortable position, with drinks and a call bell available as necessary**
Ensures patient comfort

(10) **Report the ECG to the nursing and medical team for review and interpretation. Ensure ECG filed correctly following interpretation**
Maintains patient safety and accurate records

(11) **Set alarm limits in line with patient's condition**
To ensure appropriate monitoring

(12) **Ensure cardiac monitor set to display lead II (Default Lead)**
To ensure continuous monitoring is enabled

Source: Menzies-Gow (2018)

References

Menzies-Gow, E. (2018) 'How to record a 12-lead electrocardiogram', *Nursing Standard*, 33(2): 38-42.

RESUSCITATION

EMILY MARRON AND SOPHIE NEWCOMBE

☑ Before you start

You must keep up to date with the latest guidelines available from the Resuscitation Council UK and attend regular training as per your organisation's policy. Only perform advanced airway manoeuvres once you have had the specific training and are competent to do so.

Source: Resuscitation Council UK (2015) guidelines. Available at: www.resus.org.uk

☑ Essential equipment

Below is the recommended equipment for the cardiac resuscitation trolley/bag in both primary care and acute hospitals. Equipment will vary depending on local policy and practitioner skill set.

- Personal protective equipment, sharps container, clinical waste bag
- Pocket mask with oxygen port
- Self-inflating bag-valve-mask (BVM) with reservoir with clear face masks, sizes 3, 4 and 5
- Oxygen cylinder (with key if appropriate)
- Portable suction with Yankauer sucker and soft suction catheters
- Oropharyngeal airways (OPA), sizes 2, 3 and 4
- Nasopharyngeal airways (NPA), sizes 6 and 7, and lubrication gel
- Magill forceps
- Stethoscope
- Blood glucose analyser
- Automated external defibrillator (AED)/manual defibrillator with adhesive pads, razors and tuff cut scissors

In-Hospital Advanced Life Support:

- Supraglottic airway device with syringes, lubrication and ties
- Tracheal tubes (ETT), cuffed, sizes 6, 7 and 8
- Tracheal tube introducer (stylet)
- Laryngoscope handles (x2) and blades (sizes 3 and 4) with spare batteries and bulbs (if applicable)
- Waveform capnography
- Intravenous cannulae (selection of sizes) and 2% chlorhexidine/alcohol wipes, tourniquets, cannula dressings and blood sample tubes
- Intravenous infusion set
- Selection of needles and syringes including arterial blood gas (ABG) syringe
- Intra-osseous access device
- Central venous access – Seldinger kit, full barrier precautions and skin preparation (2% chlorhexidine/alcohol)
- Ultrasound/echocardiography
- Cardiorespiratory arrest record forms for patient records, audit forms, DNACPR forms and advanced life support (ALS) algorithms
- Cardiac arrest drugs (see Resuscitation Council (UK) guidance for these)
- Adrenaline 1 mg (10 ml 1:10,000) prefilled syringe x3 (1 mg for each 3-5 minutes of CPR)
- Amiodarone 300 mg prefilled syringe x1 (first dose after three defibrillation attempts)
- 0.9% sodium chloride (1000 ml)

☑ **Care-setting considerations**

Depending on your care setting, other equipment may be considered, e.g. additional cardiac arrest drugs depending on local availability/access, ligature cutters, drug antidotes, anaphylaxis medication, towel to dry/clean chest, and moving and handling equipment.

☑ **What to watch out for and action to take**

A systematic approach using an ABCDE assessment is important when assessing your patient to ensure you recognise and treat the most significant threat to life first.

A – Airway	D – Disability
B – Breathing	E – Exposure/Environment
C – Circulation	

Basic life support (BLS) with AED: step by step

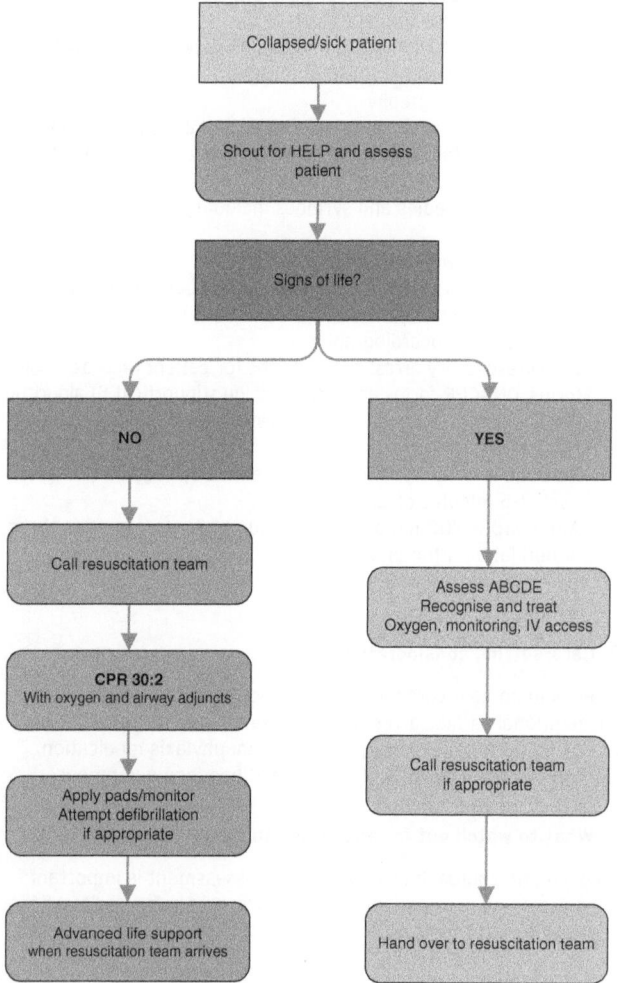

Figure 4 Resuscitation Council UK BLS algorithm

Source: Reproduced with permission of Resuscitation Council (UK)

A mnemonic often used is DRS ABC (**D**anger, **R**esponse, **S**hout, **A**irway, **B**reathing, **C**irculation).

D - Check for danger
Consider everyone's safety (including own) before approaching the patient

R - Check for a response
Gently shake their shoulders and give a command loudly in both ears, such as 'Open your eyes'. If they respond, leave them in the position in which you find them, provided there is no further danger. Reassess regularly

S - Shout for help
Call for additional help; press/pull the emergency bell if available

A - Open the patient's airway
Open the airway by turning the patient onto their back and perform either a head tilt/chin lift or jaw thrust manoeuvre (see the Basic Airway Management chapter)

B - Assess if the patient is breathing
Assess for normal breathing - look for rise and fall of the chest, listen for normal breathing sounds and feel for breath on your cheek for no more than 10 seconds

A carotid pulse check can be included at this point if competent to do so otherwise check for obvious signs of life

Not breathing and no signs of life/carotid pulse - the patient is in cardiorespiratory arrest

Get further help and send for the emergency equipment and AED
After confirming cardiorespiratory arrest you need to:

- **Dial 999 for an ambulance in the community or**
- **Dial 2222 for the adult cardiac arrest team in hospital**

C - Commence cardiac chest compressions

From the side of the patient, place the heel of one hand in the centre of the patient's chest. Place the heel of your other hand on top of your first hand and interlock your fingers

Keep your arms straight and position your shoulders vertically above the patient's chest. Press down on the sternum to a depth of 5-6 cm at a rate of 100-120 per minute for 30 compressions

After each compression, release all the pressure on the chest without losing contact between your hands and the patient's sternum

(Do not apply pressure over the patient's ribs, upper abdomen or the bottom end of the bony sternum)

A - After 30 compressions open the airway again
Use a head tilt/chin lift

B - Give two rescue breaths
Use available emergency equipment such as a pocket mask (one-person technique) or a BVM (two-person technique). Both devices should be attached to high flow oxygen if available. If no emergency equipment available undertake mouth to mouth

Pocket Mask: Open the pocket mask and place over the patient's nose and mouth. Maintain a good seal with the face mask by encircling the mask with your thumbs and index fingers whilst pressing down firmly and maintaining head tilt/chin lift. Blow steadily into the pocket mask valve whilst watching for the chest to rise. This should take 1 second as in normal breathing. Repeat to achieve two effective rescue breaths

BVM: Place the mask over the patient's nose and mouth. One person maintains a good seal with the mask as above, whilst the other squeezes the reservoir with one hand, enough to see the patient's chest rise. Repeat to achieve two effective rescue breaths

Consider inserting an airway adjunct such as an OPA or NPA (see the Basic Airway Management chapter)

Mouth to mouth resuscitation: pinch the soft part of the patient's nose closed. Allow their mouth to open but maintain head tilt/chin lift. Take a normal breath and place your lips around their mouth, ensuring a good seal. Blow steadily into the mouth while watching for the chest to rise, taking about 1 second as in normal breathing; this is an effective rescue breath. Maintaining head tilt and chin lift, take your mouth away from the patient and watch for the chest to fall. Repeat to achieve two effective rescue breaths

Do not interrupt compressions by more than 10 seconds to deliver these two breaths

C - Continue cardiac compressions
Continue with chest compressions and rescue breaths at a ratio of 30:2. If you are untrained or unable to provide rescue breaths, give continuous chest compressions only at a rate of 100-120/minute

Once an AED arrives switch it on and follow the spoken/visual instructions
Attach the adhesive pads to the patient's bare chest (remove/cut clothing if required). If you have extra help ensure BLS continues whilst the adhesive pads are attached. Ensure that nobody is touching the patient whilst the AED is analysing the rhythm

If a shock is indicated, ensure that nobody is touching the patient and oxygen is removed before delivering a safe shock by pressing the illuminated button

Immediately recommence chest compressions at a ratio of 30:2 breaths for 2 minutes

Not all cardiac arrest rhythms are shockable. If no shock is indicated, immediately recommence chest compressions 30:2 for 2 minutes as directed by the AED

Do not interrupt CPR until the following:

- An experienced health professional tells you to stop
- You become exhausted
- The patient is waking up, moving, opening eyes and breathing normally

Source: Adapted from Resuscitation Council (UK) (2015)

☑ **Helpful hints**

- In the first few minutes after cardiac arrest, a patient may be taking infrequent, ineffective slow, noisy gasps. Do not confuse agonal breaths with normal breathing.
- If the chest does not rise on the first rescue breath reposition the mask and ensure adequate seal and head tilt/chin lift.
- Well-fitting dentures if present should be kept in as this helps create a good seal.
- Attempt no more than two rescue breaths each time as this delays chest compression.
- Avoid rapid/forceful breaths when giving rescue breaths.
- If there is a risk of cervical spine injury use a jaw thrust.
- Close proximity to your patient, using your upper body weight improves chest compressions.
- Chest compressions are tiring. Aim to swap every 2 minutes if possible.
- Minimise interruptions to chest compressions (no longer than 5 seconds).
- Continue chest compressions whilst the AED is charging.
- Aim to deliver the first shock within 3 minutes.
- Do not place the adhesive pads on a wet chest, over any jewellery, medication patches or implanted devices, or deliver the shock in a highly flammable area.

Introduction to advanced life support (ALS)

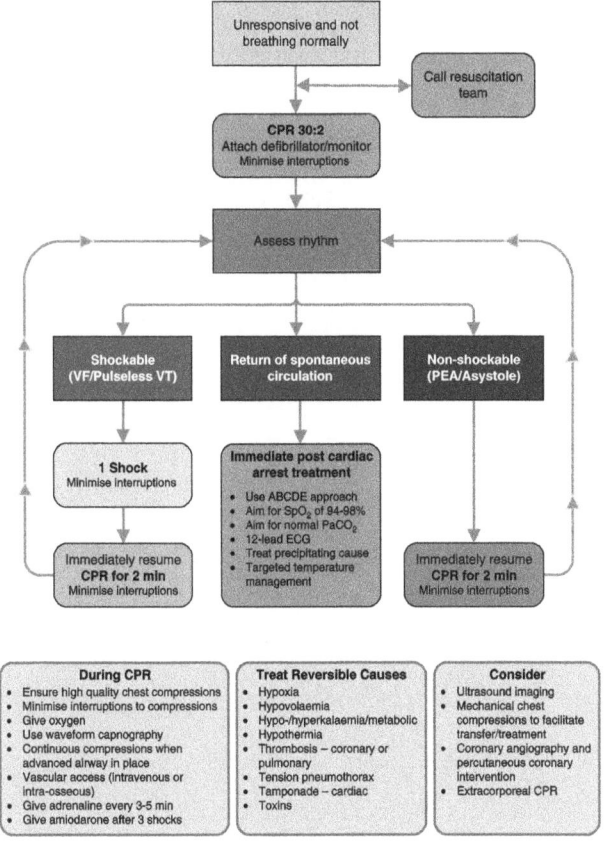

Figure 5 Resuscitation Council UK ALS algorithm

VF-ventricular fibrillation, VT-ventricular tachycardia, PEA-pulseless electrical activity

Source: Reproduced with permission of the Resuscitation Council (UK)

Once expert help arrives advanced life support commences, which includes in addition to BLS: advanced airway management, vascular access, administration of cardiac arrest drugs, and the identification and correction of reversible factors. The ALS algorithm provides a standardised approach to the management of adult patients in cardiac arrest.

References

Resuscitation Council (UK) (2015) *Resuscitation Guidelines 2015*. London: Resuscitation Council (UK).

NEUROLOGICAL EXAMINATION

WINNIE MCGARRY AND CAROLINE MACCALLUM

☑ What is normal?

Neurological examination should be performed when there is any change in the patient's neurological status. Changes can be rapid and sudden or may develop over time depending on the underlying injury.

Accurate neurological assessment is fundamental to plan appropriate patient care, and the frequency of the observations will depend on the patient's condition, diagnosis and pathology.

Neurological assessment is essential to:

- provide a baseline for observations
- monitor any changes in a patient's condition
- monitor neurological status following trauma or a neurological procedure
- aid diagnosis and establish severity of injury
- detect life-threatening situations (Dougherty and Lister, 2015).

The student nurse should be vigilant when assessing neurological observations and report any changes immediately.

Glasgow Coma Scale (GCS)

The GCS is a universal communication tool for reporting severity and outcome. This is a more detailed and complex assessment of a person's level of consciousness. Consciousness can be considered as a state of being aware of oneself and the environment and is dependent on arousability and awareness. Awareness requires an intact cerebral cortex to enable interpretation of sensory input and respond appropriately.

Neurological function is assessed in detail by observing these three elements:

1   conscious level
2   pupil size and reaction to light
3   limb assessment (motor and sensory function).

Vital signs are not included within the overall score but are required to be monitored along with neurological assessment.

The three elements above are assigned a score which results from the assessment of responses to different stimuli, and the best response is always recorded. The greater the stimulus that is required to elicit a response from the patient, the higher the likelihood of a deterioration in function.

Each response is given a potential score of 3-15. A score of 15 signifies that the patient is fully alert and responsive. A score of 3 (lowest possible) signifies that the patient is unconscious.

1   Conscious level

AVPU is a simple and quick assessment scale that can be used to rapidly assess an individual's conscious level and is used to communicate an accurate level of responsiveness to staff in a clear and understandable manner. AVPU is used to assess the patients' responses to:

Alertness

Voice

Pain

Unresponsive

It must be noted, however, that the AVPU scale does not record the subtle changes in an individual's mental state which may be an early sign that a person's condition is deteriorating. There is a significant difference between a person who is Alert and a person who is only responsive to Voice.

2 Pupil size and reaction to light

It is important to monitor pupillary reaction carefully as part of all neurological examinations, as opening of the eyes indicates arousal, which indicates brain activity, as control of the eyes is located in the brainstem.

Pupils should be assessed for:

- size, shape, equality and reaction to light (reactive, fixed, unreactive)

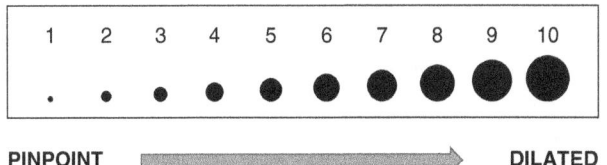

PINPOINT   **DILATED**

Figure 6   Pupil size - pinpoint to dilated

- position of the eyes: upwards or downwards
- movement: conjugate (moving together) or dysconjugate (not moving together).

Eyes should be assessed as opening:

- spontaneously
- in response to speech
- in response to pain
- no eye opening.

Note: If eyes are swollen or closed due to injury or trauma and the person is not able to open them, this should be recorded as CLOSED with a 'C'. Forcing the eye open may cause further trauma and should be avoided.

3 Limb assessment (motor and sensory function)

Motor function on both sides of the body must be monitored by assessing all four limbs. Reduced movement can be as a result of damage to the motor nervous system. This assessment takes into consideration muscle strength, tone, coordination, reflexes and any abnormal movements.

☑ Essential equipment checklist

- Alcohol hand rub
- Pen torch
- Vital signs monitoring equipment - BP, pulse, respirations and temperature
- GCS chart

☑ Care-setting considerations

Depending on the environment, i.e. within a community area, it may not always be possible to have all the equipment available to undertake a full neurological assessment such as GCS. However, many of the components can still be monitored, which will give a clear indication of the patient's physiological condition until help arrives and more equipment is available.

AVPU can be applied to all patients within any setting. However, if the patient has a reduced level of consciousness (anything less than Alert) this will require a more detailed neurological assessment using GCS.

☑ What to watch out for and action to take

When performing a full neurological assessment, if you have concerns or note any changes in the patient's level of consciousness then you must immediately report these to your mentor or registered nurse.

If trauma injury is suspected then always consider there may be a spinal injury before undertaking any interventions, cervical spine should be immobilised.

☑ Helpful hints

- Hand hygiene must be performed before touching a patient, before clean/aseptic procedures, after body fluid exposure/risk, after touching a patient and after touching a patient's surroundings.
- Equipment must be cleaned every time it is used, according to relevant policy.

Neurological examination: step by step

(1) **The first step of any procedure is to introduce yourself to the patient, explain the procedure and gain their consent to perform observations (whether conscious or not)**
It is important, as far as possible, to ensure that the patient understands the procedure and gives their consent (NMC, 2013). In the case of patients who are unable to provide consent because they are unconscious, advice should be sought from your practice educator or another registered nurse

(2) **Wash your hands with soap and water before you undertake clinical assessment. Apron and gloves should only be worn if appropriate**
Consider the individual patient situation and the risk presented and minimise the risk of cross-contamination

(3) **Observe the patient without speech or touch**
To assess eye opening as part of the GCS and level of consciousness as part of the AVPU (Fairley et al., 2005; RCP, 2012)

(4) **Talk to the patient**
Note whether they are alert and giving their full attention or restless, lethargic and drowsy. Ask the patient who they are, where they are and what day, month and year it is. Also ask them to give details about their family. Ensure that you ask the same questions consistently as this will give you a clearer indication of the patient's condition as you will be able to note any changes in their response. Ideally (and for the same reason), the assessment should be carried out by the same nurse/healthcare professional. In addition, when there is a change of shift, the assessment should be carried out by the attending healthcare professional and the person taking over the assessment of the patient
To establish whether the patient's level of consciousness is deteriorating. If the patient is becoming disorientated, changes will occur in this order:
Disorientation as to **time**, **place** and **person** (Aucken and Crawford, 1998)

5 Ask the patient to squeeze and release your fingers (both sides should be assessed) and then to stick out their tongue or raise their eyebrows
To evaluate motor responses and to ensure that the responses are equal and are not reflexive (Fairley et al., 2005)

6 If the patient does not respond, apply painful stimuli
Responses grow less purposeful as the patient's level of consciousness deteriorates. The patient may no longer localise to pain and respond to it in a purposeful way, as the condition worsens

7 Note the patient's BEST response and record this accurately
Record what stimulus was applied, where, how much pressure was required to elicit a response and how the patient responded
Accurate recording will enable continuity of assessment and comply with NMC guidelines (NMC, 2010)

8 Ask the patient to extend both hands and to squeeze your fingers as firmly as possible. Compare the grip and strength to assess
Record best arm response in GCS chart to reflect best outcome

9 Shield the patient's eyes with your hand or dim any external bright light (Fairley and Pearce, 2006a)
To allow accurate monitoring of pupil reaction

10 Ask the patient to open their eyes. If they are unable to open them for themselves, then hold their eyelids open one at a time: note size, shape and equality of both pupils
To assess and compare pupil size, shape and equality as an indicator of brain injury. Normal pupils are round, equal in size and reactive to light (Fairley et al., 2005)

11 Hold each eyelid open one at a time and shine a bright light into each. You should start from the corner of the outer eye and move slowly inwards towards the pupil. The light should cause the pupil to constrict and then brisk pupil dilation should occur when the light source is removed
To assess pupillary reflex (Fairley et al., 2005)

12 Hold both eyelids open but only shine light into one eye. Both pupils should still constrict immediately to light followed by brisk dilation when light removed
To compare both pupils and reactions (Fairley et al., 2005)

13 Record size and reactions of both pupils accurately on the observation chart, indicating brisk/sluggish/no reaction
Accurate recording and documentation will ensure continuity of assessment and compliance with NMC guidelines (NMC, 2010)

14 Record any unusual eye movements, for example deviation to the side or nystagmus
To assess cranial nerve damage

15 Measure and record the patient's respiration rate, pattern and movement
Respirations are controlled by different parts of the brain, therefore in brain injury (or disease), changes can be apparent with respirations (Jevon and Ewens, 2007)

16 Measure and record the patient's temperature regularly
The temperature-regulating centre is in the hypothalamus, therefore if damaged can result in abnormal temperature changes (Adam and Osborne, 2005)

17 Measure and record the patient's pulse and blood pressure regularly
To assess for signs of raised intracranial pressure. Hypertension and bradycardia are usually late signs and develop after there is a deterioration in the patient's conscious level (Tortora and Derrickson, 2011)

18 Ask the patient to close their eyes and hold their arms out straight in front of them, palms upwards, for 20-30 seconds. Document any weakness or drift
To assess for any limb weakness or drift (Waterhouse, 2005)

19 While standing in front of the patient with your hands extended, ask the patient to push and pull against your hands. Ask the patient to lie flat, place the patient's leg with knee flexed and foot flat on bed, then ask them to

keep their foot flat as you attempt to extend their leg. Next ask the patient to straighten their leg while you offer resistance to this
To assess arm and leg strength, to test flexion and extension in their limbs when asking them to push and pull against your resistance (Waterhouse, 2005)

(20) Observe as you ask the patient to flex and extend all limbs
To check muscle tone

(21) Ask the patient to stay lying flat, place your hand under their knee, raise and flex it. Tap the patellar tendon, and note the response (both legs)
To test the deep tendon knee-jerk reflex

(22) Stroke the lateral aspect of the sole of the patient's foot (both feet). If an abnormal response (Babinski's response), the big toe will dorsiflex while other toes will fan out
To test for upper motor neurone lesion

(23) Ask the patient to turn their hand over and back several times, noting coordination. Ask the patient to rapidly touch the back of their fingers with their thumb. Then ask the patient to touch their nose with one of their fingers several times, then repeat this instruction asking them to close their eyes
To test hand and arm/cerebellar function and coordination, dominant hand should naturally perform better

(24) Record and document all findings on the patient's observation chart. Do not be influenced by previous observations – document what you see as the patient's condition can improve/deteriorate rapidly
To ensure continuity of care and comply with NMC guidelines (2010)

(25) Immediately report any abnormal findings or changes to nursing and medical staff
To prevent deterioration and ensure rapid intervention

Wash your hands with soap and water and dry
To minimise the risk of cross-infection

 Clean equipment after use
To prevent cross-infection

Source: Adam and Osborne (2005); Aucken and Crawford (1998); Dougherty and Lister (2015); Fairley et al. (2005); Fairley and Pearce (2006a, 2006b); Fuller (2008); Jevon and Ewens (2007); McLernon and Fairley (2015); NICE (2017); NMC (2010, 2013); RCP (2012); Teasdale et al. (2014); Tortora and Derrickson (2011); Waterhouse (2005)

References

Adam, S.K. and Osborne, S. (2005)*Critical Care Nursing: Science and Practice*, 2nd edn. Oxford: Oxford University Press.

Aucken, S. and Crawford, B. (1998) 'Neurological assessment', in Guerrero, D. (ed.) *Neuro-oncology for Nurses*. London: Whurr, pp. 29-65.

Dougherty, L. and Lister, S.E. (eds) (2015) *The Royal Marsden Manual of Clinical Nursing Procedures*, 9th edn. Chichester: Wiley-Blackwell.

Fairley, D. and Pearce, A. (2006a) 'Assessment of consciousness: Part one', *Nursing Times*, *102*(4): 26-7.

Fairley, D. and Pearce, A. (2006b) 'Assessment of consciousness: Part two', *Nursing Times*, *102*(5): 26-7.

Fairley, D., Timothy, J., Donaldson-Hugh, M., Stone, M., Warren, D. and Cosgrove, J. (2005) 'Using a coma scale to assess patient consciousness levels', *Nursing Times*, *101*(25): 38-41.

Fuller, G. (2008) *Neurological Examination Made Easy*, 4th edn. Edinburgh: Churchill Livingstone.

Jevon, P. and Ewens, B. (2007) *Monitoring the Critically Ill Patient*. Oxford: Blackwell Science Limited.

National Institute for Health and Care Excellence (NICE) (2017) *Head Injury: Assessment and Early Management*. CG176. Available at: www.nice.org.uk/Guidance/CG176 (accessed 16 December 2018).

Nursing and Midwifery Council (NMC) (2010) *Record Keeping: Guidance for Nurses and Midwives*. London: NMC.

Nursing and Midwifery Council (NMC) (2013) *Consent*. London: NMC.

Royal College of Physicians (RCP) (2012) *National Early Warning Score (NEWS). Standardising the Assessment of Acute-Illness Severity in the NHS.* London: RCP. Available at: www.rcplondon.ac.uk/projects/outputs/national-early-warning-score-news-2 (accessed 16 December 2018).

Teasdale, G., Maas, A., Lecky, F., Manley, G., Stochetti, N. and Murray, G. (2014) 'The Glasgow Coma Scale at 40 years: still standing the test of time', *The Lancet Neurology, 13*: 844-54.

Tortora, G.J. and Derrickson, B.H. (2011) *Principles of Anatomy and Physiology*, 13th edn. Hoboken, NJ: John Wiley & Sons.

Waterhouse, C. (2005) 'The Glasgow Coma Scale and other neurological observations', *Nursing Standard, 19*(33): 55-64; quiz 66-7.

MEDICINES ADMINISTRATION

WINNIE MCGARRY AND CAROLINE MACCALLUM

Safety principles

All nurses adhere to the Nursing and Midwifery Council (NMC) *The Code: Professional Standards of Practice and Behaviour for Nurses and Midwives* (NMC, 2018) and *Standards for Medicines Management* (NMC, 2010), which outlines the responsibilities on medicines administration for registered nurses and midwives. Local policies and procedures are also in place to guide nurses and midwives on how to administer medicines safely.

Before medicines administration, the nurse must always consider the key principles and reflect on the five Rights:

Right **person;** Right **medicine**; Right **dose**; Right **route**; Right **time**

The patient's medicine chart must be clearly legible with full patient identifying information – patient's name, date of birth, patient's unique identifying NHS number, name of consultant caring for the patient and area of care.

Also, to be reviewed on medicine chart and confirmed with patient: prescription clear and legible, indications/contraindications/side-effects/dosage/route/frequency and time to be administered/any known allergies or sensitivities to medication/has medicine already been administered.

The British National Formulary (BNF) is a useful resource and should be referred to before medicines are administered, to ensure all the required information is checked (British Medical Association and Royal Pharmaceutical Society, 2014).

☑ Before you start

Remember the common steps for all care delivered to assist patients. It is important to involve the patient in all decisions and allow choices - their wishes should be always be priority.

☑ Essential equipment

- Medicine administration chart
- Medicine to be administered
- Medicine pot (to take the medicine to the patient in)
- Jug of water and clean glass
- Bactericidal alcohol hand gel

☑ Care-setting considerations

Medications can be administered in all care settings.

☑ Field-specific considerations

When caring for a patient with a learning disability, it is important to be aware of their level of understanding so that consent and cooperation can be gained. You will need to allow time to explain and inform the patient about their medicine and ensure their understanding. Some people living with a learning disability will be able to manage their medications while others may require support.

Patients who have mental health problems or those with a learning disability may not understand the relevance of taking their medication. They may therefore withhold consent and you may need to refer to the Mental Capacity Act 2005 and best interest. It is your responsibility to ensure that any medication given has been taken, whilst being cognisant of hiding or stockpiling medication.

☑ What to watch out for and action to take

- Ensure you understand the therapeutic effects of the medicine you are administering: normal dosage, side-effects, cautions, interactions and contraindications before you administer a medication to your patient. Always refer to the BNF to confirm this required information prior to administration.
- Note the effectiveness of the medicine post-administration: for example, pain relieved, nausea reduced.

- Always report any concerns and reactions to your mentor or another registered nurse. All reactions must be reported and treated immediately.
- Please check all packaging before opening: expiry date, packaging undamaged.
- Observe the patient for any adverse effects of the medication being administered and familiarise yourself with how to respond if a patient has an anaphylactic reaction.

☑ **Helpful hints**

- Gloves and aprons must be worn if contact with blood/body fluids/excreta is anticipated, or the patient is in isolation.
- Hand hygiene must be performed before touching a patient, before clean/aseptic procedures, after body fluid exposure/risk, after touching a patient and after touching a patient's surroundings.
- Sharps should be disposed of following local policy. Any waste must be disposed of effectively within the appropriate clinical waste bag and according to local policies.

Administering medicines: step by step

Introduce yourself to the patient, explain the procedure and gain consent
Fully informed consent may not always be possible if the patient is a child, has mental health problems or has learning disabilities. To alleviate fear and anxiety, every effort should be made to explain the procedure in terms that the patient can understand. In the case of patients who are unable to provide consent because they are unconscious, advice should be sought from your practice educator or another registered nurse

Check patient identification by asking full name and date of birth. Check information is consistent with identification bracelet if in a hospital or care environment setting
To ensure the correct medication is given to the correct patient

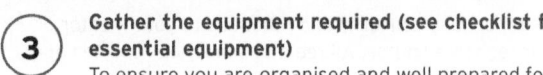

3 **Gather the equipment required (see checklist for essential equipment)**
To ensure you are organised and well prepared for the procedure

4 **Wash hands with bactericidal soap and water before you undertake the procedure and adhere to your local personal protective equipment policy. Check hands for any visibly broken skin and cover with a waterproof dressing**
To minimise the risk of contamination and infection

5 **Take all the equipment to the patient and ensure that the patient is in a comfortable position, either sitting on a chair or resting on a bed**
Promotes patient comfort and reduces anxiety

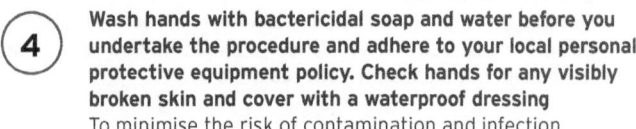

Common drug groups

Routes:

- **Intravenous (IV)**

Medications can be administered intravenously by bolus injection (small volume over shorter period) or by an intermittent or continuous infusion (larger volume which must be administered over a longer period). Student nurses are usually only allowed to give drugs via the intramuscular, subcutaneous or intradermal injection routes.

- **Per rectum (PR)**

Medications can be administered into the rectum and are absorbed through the rectal mucosa. They may also be given for topical use: for haemorrhoids, to stimulate the bowel to work and to encourage defaecation. Many medications can be administered rectally, if the patient is unable to take medication orally. Can be administered in liquid or solid (suppository) form.

- **Per vagina (PV)**

Medicines can be inserted into the vagina, for topical use only. The medication is normally inserted using an applicator high into the vagina. It can also be delivered as a pessary (vaginal suppository) or a cream.

- **Sublingual (SL)/buccal**

Sublingual medication should be placed under the tongue.
Buccal medication should be placed between the top lip and gum.

- **Nasogastric (NG)/percutaneous endoscopic gastrostomy (PEG)**

At times there may be some patients who are unable to take
medication orally. Some medicines may be administered via a
nasogastric (NG) tube or percutaneous endoscopic gastrostomy
(PEG) tube directly into the stomach. Medicines administered via
these routes must be given in appropriate soluble or liquid form.

- **Transdermal**

Transdermal medication is administered from an impregnated,
adhesive patch. The medication is slowly released from the patch
and absorbed through the skin: this ensures that the medicine is
delivered through a steady blood level. The patch should be placed
on an area of clean, dry skin which has been assessed and is in good
condition.

- **Infusion pump (subcutaneous)**

Infusion pumps are commonly used to administer medications, fluids
and nutrients intravenously and subcutaneously. Infusion pumps can
administer larger volumes of medications or fluids, or very small
volumes can be administered accurately at varying speeds. The main
types of infusion pumps are: volumetric, ambulatory volumetric,
syringe infusion and patient-controlled analgesia.

Using patient group directions (PGDs)

Patient group directions (PGDs) provide a legal framework that
allows supply and/or administration of a specified medicine/s, by
named, authorised, registered health professionals to a pre-defined
group of patients. These are written instructions that permit supply
or administration without the need for a prescription or an
instruction from a prescriber to pre-defined groups of patients
needing treatment or prophylaxis for a condition described in the
PGD. However, using a PGD is not a form of prescribing. There are
specific policies and processes in place by organisations to ensure
that when PGDs are used they are legal, appropriate and that

governance arrangements are in place (RCN, 2017). It should be noted that there are differences between the home nations. (NES 2015).

Anaphylaxis management

Ensure that you establish if the patient has any allergies, and also ensure that you are familiar with the importance of knowing how to respond to anaphylaxis.

Source: British Medical Association and Royal Pharmaceutical Society (2014); Dougherty and Lister (2015); NMC (2018); RCN (2017)

References

British Medical Association and Royal Pharmaceutical Society (2014) *British National Formulary 67*. London: Pharmaceutical Press.

Dougherty, L. and Lister, S.E. (eds) (2015) *The Royal Marsden Manual of Clinical Nursing Procedures*, 9th edn. Chichester: Wiley-Blackwell.

Mental Capacity Act (2005) Available at: www.legislation.gov.uk/ukpga/2005/9/pdfs/ukpga_20050009_en.pdf (accessed 10 August 2018).

NHS Education for Scotland *Patient Group Directions*. Available at: www.nes.scot.nhs.uk/education-and-training/by-theme-initiative/prescribing-and-patient-group-direction/ (accessed 16 December 2018).

Nursing and Midwifery Council (NMC) (2010) London: NMC. Available at: www.nmc.org.uk/ globalassets/sitedocuments/nmc-publications/nmc-code.pdf

Nursing and Midwifery Council (NMC) (2018) *The Code: Professional Standards of Practice and Behaviour for Nurses, Midwives and Nursing Associates*. London: NMC. Available at: www.nmc.org.uk/globalassets/sitedocuments/nmc-publications/nmc-code.pdf (accessed 31 October 2018).

Royal College of Nursing (RCN) (2017) *Patient Specific Directions (PSDs) and Patient Group Directions (PGDs)*. London: RCN. Available at: www.rcn.org.uk/clinical-topics/medicines-optimisation/specialist-areas/patient-specific-directions-and-patient-group-directions (accessed 16 December 2018).

BOWEL SOUNDS

WINNIE MCGARRY AND CAROLINE MACCALLUM

☑ What is normal?

Bowel sounds are the noises made by the movement of the intestines as they push food through the gastrointestinal tract - this is normal. Auscultation is the process by which we are able to listen to bowel sounds using a stethoscope. The intestines are hollow, therefore the sounds we hear are echoed through the abdomen. If we are familiar with 'normal' bowel sounds, we are able to detect 'abnormal' changes in bowel sounds using auscultation.

☑ Before you start

Review the anatomy and physiology of the gastrointestinal tract. It is useful to divide the abdomen into four quadrants. It is important that you auscultate **over all four quadrants** and that you are aware of what you are listening and feeling for when assessing bowel sounds.

No bowel sounds: Auscultate over the quadrant for at least 5 minutes to confirm (e.g. no bowel sounds can be a sign of paralytic ileus).

Hypoactive bowel sounds: A sign that intestinal activity has slowed. This may include a reduction in the loudness, tone or regularity of the sounds and register one every 3 to 5 minutes (e.g. constipation, may also be caused by some opiates, anticholinergics and phenothiazines).

Hyperactive bowel sounds: Excessive bowel sounds that can sometimes be heard without using a stethoscope. Often heard before a blockage (for example, anything that is increasing peristalsis, e.g. immediately following a meal, cramping, stomach upset, inflammatory bowel disease, infectious enteritis).

No bowel sounds after an episode of hyperactive bowel sounds: May be a sign of intestinal rupture or strangulation of the bowel and necrosis of bowel tissue.

☑ **Essential equipment**

- Stethoscope

☑ **Care-setting considerations**

It is not always possible to have a quiet area to carry out this examination; however, where possible the noise level should be at a minimum. It is important to ensure privacy during the examination.

☑ **What to watch out for and action to take**

While carrying out this examination, you should also assess:

- thorough medical history (including diet and fluid intake and condition of the mouth)
- any signs of persistent altered bowel habit (constipation, diarrhoea)
- any signs or complaints of abdominal pain
- any signs of abdominal distention
- any signs of flatus or absence of flatus
- any bleeding from the back passage (note the colour of the blood passed)
- the general condition of the patient
- their neurological condition – are they alert and responsive?
- are they agitated?
- any signs or complaints of pain or discomfort
- the patient's relatives'/carers' views – for example, saying that their condition is 'not quite right' or they 'don't feel well'.

The outcome of this assessment should be shared with medical staff and reported in the patient's record.

- Hand hygiene must be performed before touching a patient, before clean/aseptic procedures, after body fluid exposure/risk, after touching a patient and after touching a patient's surroundings.
- Gently warm hands before touching the patient.
- Equipment must be cleaned as identified by the relevant policy every time it is used.

Assessing bowel sounds: step by step

The first step of any procedure is to introduce yourself to the patient, explain the procedure and gain their consent
Fully informed consent may not always be possible if the patient is a child, has mental health problems or has learning disabilities; even in these circumstances, however, every effort should be made to explain the procedure in terms that the patient can understand. In the case of patients who are unable to provide consent because they are unconscious, advice should be sought from your practice educator or another registered nurse

Gather the equipment required (identified above). Ensure stethoscope is clean and in working order
To optimise accurate auscultation of the abdomen. Reduces the chance of infection and maintains patient and nurse safety

Clear sufficient space within the environment
Enables clear access for the patient and the nurse to safely carry out the examination

Wash your hands with soap and water before you undertake clinical assessment
Apron and gloves should only be worn if appropriate. Consider the individual patient situation and the risk presented

5 Ask the patient if they wish to have the curtains drawn for privacy or to be in a separate room
Maintains patient privacy, dignity and comfort

6 The patient should be in a supine position with head and knees supported. In an emergency situation where the patient has collapsed or is acutely unwell, the assessment should be taken wherever the patient is situated
Promotes patient comfort and reduce anxiety

7 Observe the abdomen for signs of symmetry. Is the abdomen bloated or bulging in any part? Is there any obvious signs of peristaltic movement?
To identify potential visual abnormalities before auscultation

8 Using the stethoscope to auscultate the abdomen, start at the right lower quadrant (RLQ) and move clockwise to follow the normal movement of peristalsis. This part of the assessment must be carried out before palpation
Palpation stimulates peristalsis, therefore auscultation is carried out first to listen for hyperactive, hypoactive or no bowel activity. Helps put the patient at ease and encourages cooperation

9 Gently palpate the abdomen using your fingertips
This will help you to identify crepitus of the abdominal wall, a sign of gas or fluid within the subcutaneous tissues. It may also identify any irregularities of the abdominal wall (e.g. hernia, tumour) and help identify areas of tenderness. Helps put the patient at ease and encourages cooperation

10 Starting at the RLQ and moving clockwise to follow the normal movement of peristalsis, place the flat of your hand on the abdominal wall and apply firm steady pressure to palpate the abdomen
This will help you further to identify any irregularities of the abdominal wall (e.g. hernia, tumour, adhesions, obstruction) and help identify areas of tenderness

11 Leave the patient comfortable
Promotes patient comfort and reduces anxiety

12 **Document date and time of examination and any concerns noted in patient's records immediately**
Maintains patient safety and accurate records

Source: Ball et al. (2015); Dougherty and Lister (2015); NMC (2018)

References

Ball, J.W., Dains, J.E., Flynn, J.A., Solomon, B.S. and Stewart, R.W. (2015) *Siedel's Guide to Physical Examination*, 8th edn. St Louis, MO: Elsevier Mosby.

Dougherty, L. and Lister, S.E. (eds) (2015) *The Royal Marsden Manual of Clinical Nursing Procedures*, 9th edn. Chichester: Wiley-Blackwell.

Nursing and Midwifery Council (NMC) (2018) The Code: Professional Standards of Practice and Behaviour for Nurses, Midwives and Nursing Associates. London: NMC. Available at: www.nmc.org.uk/globalassets/sitedocuments/nmc-publications/nmc-code.pdf (accessed 31 October 2018).

GASTRIC ASPIRATION
SUE MCGROUTHER AND JULIE ORR

☑ **Before you start**

The insertion of a wide bore nasogastric (NG) tube facilitates the drainage of fluid or gas in acutely ill patients with intestinal obstruction or ileus. These are used short term since they can cause nasal irritation/damage (Endacott et al., 2009). Gastric fluids can be allowed to drain freely or intermittently.

☑ **Essential equipment**

- Radio opaque wide bore NG tube with spigot
- Lubricant in accordance with the manufacturer's instructions and/or local policy
- Personal protective equipment; non-sterile gloves and apron
- Tissues and a glass of water
- Sterile water
- 50 ml and 20 ml syringes
- Non-allergenic tape
- Vomit bowl

Source: Baillie (2014)

☑ **What to watch out for and action to take**

Contraindications to NG Aspiration: Past and current medical history should be ascertained. Contraindications can include:

- complex head, face, neck or basal skull fractures/facial deformities or trauma

- upper GI pathology (Peate and Gault, 2013)
- bleeding disorders (Baillie, 2014).

Complications: Observe and assess patient throughout and following NG insertion and aspiration procedure. If there are any signs of deterioration, carry out A-E assessment and communicate with relevant members of the multidisciplinary team.

- Pulmonary aspiration
- Pneumothorax
- Cardiovascular irregularities including narrow complex tachycardia (Smith et al., 2012)
- Continuous aspiration can lead to the NG tube tip adhering to the abdominal wall

Prolonged use of a wide bore tube can lead to tube stiffening and tube perforation (Baillie, 2014)

☑ Helpful hints

- Personal protective equipment (PPE): gloves and aprons must be worn if contact with blood/body fluids/excreta is anticipated, or the patient is in isolation.
- Hand hygiene must be performed before touching a patient, before clean/aseptic procedures, after body fluid exposure/risk, after touching a patient and after touching a patient's surroundings.
- Waste should be disposed of in a clinical waste bag if appropriate.

Gastric aspiration: step by step

1 **The first step in any procedure is to introduce yourself to the patient, explain the procedure and gain consent**
Fully informed consent may not always be possible if the patient is a child, has mental health problems or has learning disabilities. To alleviate fear and anxiety, every effort should be made to explain the procedure in terms

that the patient can understand. In the case of patients who are unable to provide consent because they are unconscious, advice should be sought from your practice educator or another registered nurse

2 **Check patient identification by asking full name and date of birth. Check information is consistent with identification bracelet if in a hospital setting**
To ensure the procedure is carried out on the correct person (NHS Improvement, 2018)

3 **Gather the equipment required (see checklist for equipment required)**
To ensure you are organised and well prepared for the procedure

4 **Wash hands with bactericidal soap and water before you undertake the procedure and adhere to your local PPE policy. Check hands for any visibly broken skin, and cover with a waterproof dressing**
To minimise the risk of contamination and infection (NHS Education for Scotland, 2017)

5 **Connect either a 50 ml catheter tip syringe or suction equipment, per manufacturer's instructions or clinical guidance, to the larger, primary lumen**
Gentle suction should be applied to prevent damage to the gastric mucosa (NHS Foundation Trust, 2017)

6 **Aspirate gastric contents every 30-60 minutes initially**
Depending on the patient's condition and clinical guidance (Gallacher, 2011; Powers, 2014)

7 **Observe the volume, colour and consistency of the gastric contents**
In order to maintain accurate fluid balance and enable effective patient assessment

8 **Record assessment findings in accordance with the NMC Code (2018) and communicate findings to your mentor or trained staff**
Maintains patient safety and accurate records

9 **Observe the patient for any signs of complication from the procedure**
If there are any signs of deterioration, carry out A-E assessment and communicate with relevant members of the multidisciplinary team

10 **Discard PPE, any single-use equipment and other used materials as per local policy**
To prevent cross-infection

11 **After performing the skill, ensure the patient is comfortable with a call bell available**
To promote patient comfort

12 **Perform hand hygiene**
To minimise risk of infection (NHS Education for Scotland, 2017)

13 **Document date, time of procedure and any concerns noted in patient's records immediately**
Maintains patient safety and accurate records (NMC, 2018)

Source: Baillie (2014); Endacott et al. (2009); Gallacher (2011); NHS Education for Scotland (2017); NHS Foundation Trust (2017); NHS Improvement (2018); NMC (2018); Peate and Gault (2013); Powers (2014); Smith et al. (2012).

References

Baillie, L. (2014) *Developing Practical Nursing Skills*, 4th edn. Boca Raton, FL: Taylor Francis.

Endacott, R., Jevon, P. and Cooper, S. (2009) *Clinical Nursing Skills: Core and Advanced*. New York: Oxford University Press.

Gallacher, B. (2011) 'Small bowel obstruction', in Gallacher, B., Clarke, D. and Ketchell, A. (eds) *Nursing the Acutely Ill Adult*. Houndmills: Palgrave MacMillan.

NHS Education for Scotland (2017) *Healthcare Associated Infections: Pathway-Foundation layer*. Available at: www.nes.scot.nhs.uk/education-and-training/by-theme-initiative/healthcare-associated-infections/scottish-infection-prevention-and-control-education-pathway/pathway-foundation-layer.aspx (accessed 30 October 2018).

NHS Foundation Trust (2017) *Nasogastric Tube Management and Care*. Doncaster: Doncaster & Bassetlaw Teaching Hospital.

NHS Improvement (2018) *Recommendations from National Patient Safety Agency Alerts That Remain Relevant to the Never Events List 2018*. London: NHS Improvement.

Nursing and Midwifery Council (NMC) (2018) *The Code: Professional Standards of Practice and Behaviour for Nurses, Midwives and Nursing Associates*. London: NMC. Available at: www.nmc.org.uk/globalassets/sitedocuments/nmc-publications/nmc-code.pdf (accessed 31 October 2018).

Peate, I. and Gault, C. (2013) 'Clinical skills series 4: Nasogastric tube insertion', *British Journal of Healthcare Assistants*, 7(6): 272-7. Available at: www.magonlinelibrary.com/doi/abs/10.12968/bjha.2013.7.6.272 (accessed 31 October 2018).

Powers, J.M. (2014) 'Use of gastric decompression tubes with small-bowel feeding tubes', *Critical Care Nurse*, *34*(3): 84-5.

Smith, N.L., Park, M. and Freebairn, R. (2012) 'Case report and review-nasogastric tube complications', *Critical Care & Shock*, *15*(2): 36-42. Available at: https://pdfs.semanticscholar.org/49a2/0de94fb3d245bbdd71e5cd1e4f69f2ca7742.pdf

ENTERAL FEEDING
MARK MOLESWORTH AND MOIRA DALE

Enteral feeding involves the delivery of a supplementary or nutritionally complete feed via a tube which discharges directly into the patient's gastrointestinal system. In most cases the nutrition will enter the stomach, delivered via a nasogastric (NG) or percutaneous endoscopic gastrostomy (PEG) tube; although for some patients the tube may terminate in the duodenum or jejunum.

☑ Before you start

- Ensure you have received appropriate training in enteral feeding and are familiar with relevant policies and procedures.
- Take into consideration any contraindications, for example:
    - partial or subtotal gastrectomy
    - massive ascites
    - portal hypertension
    - peritoneal dialysis
    - active gastric pathology
    - coagulation disorders
    - sepsis
    - pyloric stenosis.

☑ Care-setting considerations

In hospital settings, sterile water is often used to flush the enteral feeding tube, although there is variation across different regions so check local policies and procedures if unsure. When flushing the enteral feeding tube in primary and community care settings, freshly drawn tap water for patients who are not immunosuppressed or cooled freshly boiled water/sterile water from a freshly opened container for patients who are immunosuppressed may be used (NICE, 2012a).

☑ What to watch out for and action to take, including complications

There can be serious clinical consequences if the enteral feed is not administered correctly.

- NEVER connect or administer enteral medicines or feed to an intravenous cannula as this is known to cause patient harm and can be fatal. Manufacturers have developed devices to prevent this occurring, including the Reverse Luer Lock™ system introduced in 2007 and more recently the ENFit™ connector (Holland, 2015). At the time of writing a phased approach is being used to introduce the ENFit™ system nationally but some areas may have old systems in place – check if unsure.
- Patients who are at high risk of fluid overload and/or depend upon concentrated feeding formula may have specific instructions for flushing the tube.
- Contamination of the enteral feed can lead to healthcare-associated infection. It is essential that infection control and prevention precautions are followed and that the feed is stored correctly, and all equipment is appropriately used, monitored and maintained (Malhi, 2017; NICE, 2012b).
- If there is pain on feeding, leakage of gastric contents or bleeding, stop the feed and seek advice from an appropriately skilled practitioner (Fletcher, 2011).

Complications

- Refeeding syndrome is a serious condition associated with severe and potentially fatal shifts in the patient's electrolyte and fluid levels. It usually occurs following the introduction or recommencement of artificial refeeding after long periods of starvation, with underweight patients and those experiencing unintentional weight loss at increased risk (NICE, 2006).
- Electrolyte/metabolic abnormalities may occur. The protocol for laboratory monitoring of nutrition support may be used for patients who are metabolically unstable or at risk of refeeding syndrome (NICE, 2006).

- Reflux and vomiting, abdominal pain/distension, diarrhoea, constipation (BAPEN, 2018)

☑ Helpful hints

- Encourage the patient to assist in the procedure if it is safe and appropriate to do so.
- After the initial tube insertion and commencement of feeding, the patient may have ongoing concerns. Communicate with the patient at each episode of care, allowing for questions to be asked whilst providing reassurance and information as appropriate.
- Remember that medication should not be added directly to the feed.
- Cultural aspects in relation to the content of the feed should be considered such as the need to accommodate halal, kosher and vegan diets.
- Hand hygiene must be performed before touching a patient, before clean/aseptic procedures, after body fluid exposure/risk, after touching a patient and after touching a patient's surroundings.

☑ Essential equipment

Ensure all packaging is intact and the equipment is within the expiry date. The following items are required:

- prescribed enteral feed at room temperature
- prescription/regimen
- pH sensitive strips/X-ray confirmation of NG tube position if applicable
- non-sterile gloves and apron
- 60 ml enteral syringe
- sterile water or fresh cooled boiled water/tap water depending upon the patient's immune status and the setting.

You may also require an extension set and adapters/connectors depending upon the circumstances.
Additional items for pump method:

- compatible enteral feeding pump
- compatible administration set (giving set)
- drip stand.

Administering the feed: step by step

Note that there are two different methods discussed, so check which one applies prior to commencing the procedure.

Preparation

(1) Introduce yourself to the patient, explain the procedure and gain consent
Fully informed consent may not always be possible if the patient is a child, has mental health problems or has learning disabilities. To alleviate fear and anxiety, every effort should be made to explain the procedure in terms that the patient can understand. In the case of patients who are unable to provide consent because they are unconscious, advice should be sought from your practice educator or another registered nurse

(2) Gather the equipment required (see checklist for equipment required)
To ensure you are organised and well prepared for the procedure

(3) Wash hands with bactericidal soap and water before you undertake the procedure and adhere to your local personal protective equipment policy. Check hands for any visibly broken skin, and cover with a waterproof dressing
To minimise the risk of contamination and infection (NHS National Services Scotland, 2012)

(4) Check the prescription is valid and that it matches the feed you intend to commence
To ensure that the correct amount of prescribed feed is administered to the patient, it is delivered at the right time of day and at the correct rate via the correct route

(5) Check patient allergies
To ensure that there are no allergies which would put the patient at risk of a reaction when the feed is commenced. Consider latex allergy

6 Gather the necessary equipment and, if required, reconstitute the feed following the manufacturer guidelines. Where possible pre-packaged, ready-to-use feeds should be used (NICE, 2012a)

To ensure the feed is made to the correct concentration and to avoid the risk of contamination of the feed

7 Ensure the procedure is carried out in an appropriate environment maintaining patient privacy and dignity throughout. Only expose the area of the body necessary to gain access to the feeding tube

To ensure patient dignity, privacy, comfort and respect is maintained throughout the procedure

8 Assess the feeding tube site for signs of infection or movement. These must be reported and documented immediately

To prevent any unnecessary complications and undue risk to the patient

9 Clean the site if necessary, using 0.9% sodium chloride solution. Dry thoroughly

To assess the site for signs of infection and to prevent contamination of the site

10 Prior to administering the nutrition ensure the abdomen is not distended and there is no tenderness or rigidity. If there are any concerns seek advice prior to proceeding

To prevent any unnecessary complications and undue risk to the patient

11 Position the patient appropriately, with the upper body at a minimum angle of 30 degrees throughout the administration of the feed

To avoid reflux of the feed whilst also reducing the risk of aspiration, which is a serious complication resulting from the entry of the contents of the gastrointestinal tract into the patient's lungs

Administration

If using the enteral pump method (bolus, intermittent or continuous feeding) with a pre-packaged feed:

1 **If feeding via an NG tube check the positioning of the tube in accordance with applicable policy and guidelines**
To ensure the tube is situated in the stomach and the feed is delivered safely

2 **Open the enteral feeding tube and flush it with 30-50 ml sterile water using the 60 ml enteral syringe. Close the enteral feeding tube once finished**
To prevent blockage of the tube

3 **Check the expiry date of the feed and shake the container to mix the contents**
To ensure the feed is safe to deliver and that the contents are evenly dispersed

4 **Close the administration set then spike the feed container using a non-touch technique**
To attach the feed to the administration set whilst reducing the risk of contamination of the feed

5 **Hang the container on the drip-stand and squeeze the administration set drip chamber so that it fills to the required level (do not overfill the drip chamber)**
To ensure the administration set is ready to be primed correctly, reducing the likelihood of subsequent problems and avoiding the introduction of air into the line

6 **Depending upon the model of pump, prime the administration set manually or use the appropriate function on the pump. Take care to minimise the amount of air in the line**
To introduce the feed along the entire length of the line by replacing all the air

7 **Connect the administration set to the enteral feeding tube**
To allow delivery of the feed. Be careful not to contaminate the open ends of the administration set and the enteral feeding tube during this stage

Label the administration set with the date of commencement. The administration set should be changed every 24 hours
This will ensure the administration set is not utilised for longer than is acceptable, providing information to all staff in relation to when the administration set is due to be replaced. This measure reduces the risk of contamination and the potential for patient infection

Programme the pump to the appropriate mode and set the volume and rate in accordance with the prescription
To ensure the delivery of the prescribed feed exactly matches the prescription

Ensure the administration set and enteral feeding tube are open and start the pump
To allow delivery of the feed

Monitor the administration of the feed as appropriate
To observe for any patient complications which need to be assessed and managed whilst responding to any equipment issues promptly

Flush the enteral feeding tube with 30-50 ml sterile water using the 60 ml enteral syringe once the feed has concluded
To prevent blockage of the tube

If using the gravity syringe method (bolus feeding):

If feeding via an NG tube check the positioning of the tube in accordance with applicable policy and guidelines
To ensure the tube is situated in the stomach and the feed is delivered safely

Check the expiry date of the feed and, if using a pre-packaged feed, shake the container to mix the contents
To ensure the feed is safe to deliver and that the contents are evenly dispersed

Remover the plunger from the 60 ml enteral syringe then attach it to the enteral feeding tube
To allow delivery of the feed. Be careful not to contaminate the open ends of the syringe and the enteral feeding tube during this stage

4 Add 30-50 ml sterile water to the enteral syringe and open the enteral feeding tube to flush it. Close the enteral feeding tube once finished
To prevent blockage of the tube

5 Add the feed to the enteral syringe and ensure it is above the level of the patient
To allow the feed to flow via gravity into the patient

6 Open the enteral feeding tube to allow the feed to flow using gravity
To allow the prescribed amount of feed to be delivered at the correct rate. Raising the enteral syringe will increase the flow rate and lowering it will decrease it

7 Close the enteral feeding tube if it is necessary to refill the enteral syringe, allowing it to flow again once refilled
To control the delivery of the feed whilst minimising the risk of air entering the enteral feeding tube. Avoid allowing the enteral syringe to empty completely before adding more feed

8 Flush the enteral feeding tube with 30-50 ml sterile water once the feed has concluded
To prevent blockage of the tube

9 Close the feeding tube and discard the enteral syringe, although in some settings it may be reused for up to one week. If it is to be reused, wash the enteral syringe in warm soapy water and leave to air dry
To minimise the risk of contamination of the enteral syringe

10 Unused feed should be labelled with the patient's details along with the date and time of opening. Store in a refrigerator for use up to 24 hours after opening
This will ensure the feed is discarded after the time limit for administration has passed, providing information to all staff to prevent the risk of contamination and the potential for patient infection

After the procedure:

 The patient should remain in an upright position for at least 1 hour after the administration of the enteral feed has concluded. Avoid lying the patient flat as this increases the risk of aspiration
This is another measure which reduces the risk of aspiration, which is a serious complication resulting from the entry of the contents of the gastrointestinal tract into the patient's lungs

 Ensure the patient is comfortable and able to gain assistance if required. Provide relevant information about the procedure and offer the patient opportunities to ask questions and provide feedback regarding their experience
To ensure the delivery of person-centred care to the individual patient

 Record the amount of feed administered along with details of the flushes undertaken
To ensure accurate documentation of the delivered feed and to allow careful monitoring of the patient's fluid intake where appropriate

 Complete all relevant documentation and communicate with other members of the multidisciplinary team as necessary
To ensure accurate documentation of the delivered feed, the procedure followed and any complications or problems. This step is integral to effective communication within the nursing and multidisciplinary team, promoting safety and continuity of care

 Remember that enteral tube feeding should be reviewed when the patient is established on adequate oral intake (NICE, 2006)
To ensure that the patient does not receive enteral feeding if it is not indicated

 At regular intervals, review the indications, route, risks, benefits and goals of nutrition support (NICE, 2006)
To ensure appropriate means of nutritional intake

Source: Adults with Incapacity (Scotland) Act (2000); Best (2010); BAPEN (2018); Fletcher (2011); Holland (2015); Holmes (2004); Malhi (2017); Mental Capacity Act (2005); NICE (2006, 2012a, 2012b); NMC (2010)

Acknowledgement

Jennifer McClorey, Community Nutrition Support Dietician, NHS Dumfries and Galloway.

References

Adults with Incapacity (Scotland) Act (2000) Available at: www.legislation.gov.uk/asp/2000/4/contents (accessed 1 August 2018).

Best, C. (2010) 'Introducing enteral nutrition support: ethical considerations', *Nursing Standard*, 24(37): 41-5.

British Association for Parenteral and Enteral Nutrition (BAPEN) (2018) *Enteral Feeding*. Available at: www.bapen.org.uk/nutrition-support/enteral-nutrition (accessed 14 June 2018).

Fletcher, J. (2011) 'Nutrition: Safe practice in adult enteral tube feeding', *British Journal of Nursing*, 20(19): 1234-9.

Holland, M. (2015) 'Enhancing patient safety in enteral feeding', *Nursing Times*, 111(38): 22-3.

Holmes, S. (2004) 'Enteral feeding and percutaneous endoscopic gastrostomy', *Nursing Standard*, 18(20): 41-3.

Malhi, H. (2017) 'Enteral tube feeding: Using good practice to prevent infection', *British Journal of Nursing*, 26(1): 8-14.

Mental Capacity Act (2005) Available at: www.legislation.gov.uk/ukpga/2005/9/pdfs/ukpga_20050009_en.pdf (accessed 10 August 2018).

National Institute for Health and Care Excellence (NICE) (2006) *Nutrition Support for Adults: Oral Nutrition Support, Enteral Feeding and Parenteral Nutrition*. Clinical Guideline 32. Available at: www.nice.org.uk/Guidance/cg32 (accessed 14 June 2018).

National Institute for Health and Care Excellence (NICE) (2012a) *Healthcare-Associated Infections: Prevention and Control in Primary and Community Care*. Available at: www.nice.org.uk/guidance/cg139 (accessed 12 August 2018).

National Institute for Health and Care Excellence (NICE) (2012b) *Nutrition Support in Adults*. Quality Standard 24. Available at: www.nice.org.uk/guidance/qs24 (accessed 10 July 2018).

NHS National Services Scotland (2012) National Infection Prevention and Control Manual. Available at: www.nipcm.hps.scot.nhs.uk/chapter-1-standard-infection-control-precautions-sicps/#a1069 (accessed 23 January 2019).

Nursing and Midwifery Council (NMC) (2010) *Record Keeping: Guidance for Nurses and Midwives*. London: NMC.

REMOVAL OF SUTURES AND STAPLES

FRANCINA HYATT

☑ Before you start

Always assess the wound, considering the time period for removal of sutures or staples; this will depend upon the site of the wound, underlying pathology and surgical instructions. Analgesia may need to be offered based on individual assessment and level of comfort. Seek advice from a registered clinician if the wound appears infected or if there is evidence of delayed healing.

Source: Dougherty and Lister (2015); Perry and Potter (2015)

☑ Essential equipment

- Detergent wipe to clean trolley or area for opening a dressing pack onto
- Alcohol gel or access to a hand-washing sink
- Sterile gloves and apron
- Sterile dressing pack containing a gallipot, disposable forceps, sterile field, gauze, disposable bag
- Sterile cleaning fluid and sterile syringe for irrigation, if needed
- Staple remover (if removing staples)
- Stitch cutter
- Sterile scissors
- Appropriate dressing according to holistic assessment of the patient
- Traceability system for surgical instruments (if applicable)

Source: Department of Health (2011); Dougherty and Lister (2015)

Removal of sutures or staples can be undertaken in any setting, but care must be taken to prevent contamination of the sterile field. Good patient positioning to allow easy removal and management of a possible syncope (faint) must also be considered.

☑ What to watch out for and action to take

- There are varying suture techniques which may be used according to tissue types, parts of the body and whether temporary or permanent wound closure is needed.
- Ensure you have received correct training, supervision and assessment prior to removing sutures or staples.
- Suture materials can stimulate their own inflammatory response, which should be taken into account when assessing the wound for an infection.
- Do not remove remaining sutures or staples if wound dehiscence (reopening) occurs.
- Always discard your blade and staples directly into a sharps bin after use to avoid a potential blood borne infection caused by a sharps injury.

☑ Helpful hints

- Remove any protective dressing using non-sterile gloves and whilst wearing an apron prior to starting the aseptic part of the procedure.
- Always clean away any dried blood or scabs to ensure all the sutures and staples are removed and none are missed.
- Do not lift the staple remover while squeezing the handle. If you feel resistance do not force removal, and seek advice from a registered clinician.

Source: McClelland and Nellis (1997); Pudner (2005); Pullen (2003)

Removal of suture or staples: step by step

Perform a basic patient assessment, including clinical measurement, if deemed necessary
To prepare the patient and yourself to perform the procedure

2 **Place the patient in a comfortable position, conducive to removal of the sutures or staples**
A patient may need to be lying supine or prone or in the Fowler's position (sitting up) to ensure easy access and visualisation of the wound

3 **Ask the patient if they wish to have the curtains drawn or to be in a separate room. When applicable offer to provide a chaperone**
Maintains privacy, dignity and comfort. Protects the patient and clinician if removing sutures from an intimate area of the body

4 **Check all equipment is in date and inspect packaging for rips and tears**
To ensure all equipment used is aseptic

5 **Open a dressing pack following an aseptic technique and add your stitch cutter or staple remover, cleaning solution and dressing of choice**
Reduces likelihood of contaminating sterile gloves once donned

6 **Perform hand hygiene again with alcohol gel**
To decontaminate hands prior to putting on sterile gloves

7 **Put on well-fitting sterile gloves**
This is required to maintain an aseptic technique. A healed wound may be assessed as suitable to undertake an aseptic non-touch technique; however, this is subject to individual risk assessment, local policy and current evidence

8 **Clean or irrigate the wound with a cleaning solution such as 0.9% sodium chloride, if required**
To remove dried blood or exudate ensuring good visibility of the wound

9 **Lift the suture knot to allow for the stitch cutter to cut the suture as close to the skin as possible. Use the forceps to gently pull the suture through the skin pulling towards the side that has been cut**
Gently press the skin with the side of the cutter or scissors as you remove the stitch to reduce pulling on the skin: this

will lesson pain for the patient as well. For intermittent sutures, alternate sutures should be removed to assess for signs of wound opening. Seek advice from a registered clinician as needed (Figure 7)

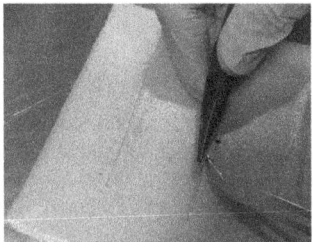

Figure 7   Suture removal

(10) **When removing staples, slide the V-shaped groove of the lower bar of the staple remover under the staple at 90 degrees whilst gently squeezing the handles of the staple remover. The staple will open; however, if the suture line is under tension, gently squeeze either side of the suture line with your free hand to reduce the tension**
Correct positioning of the staple remover is important both for patient comfort and to ensure the staple opens in a way that allows for easy removal. Always remove alternate staples to allow assessment of skin integrity (Figure 8)

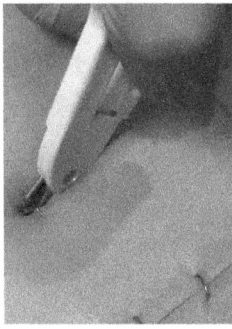

Figure 8   Staple removal

(11) **Consider application of adhesive skin tapes**
To support the tensile strength of the wound, advise the patient the adhesive skin tapes should be left in situ until they fall off by themselves

(12) **Dispose of all equipment according to local policy and NICE guidelines**
To ensure correct disposal of clinical waste

(13) **Observe and record condition of suture line, reporting any signs of infection, and assess patient's pain. Record how many sutures or staples you have removed and document this in the patient's notes**
An infected wound will need assessment for antibiotic therapy and the patient may need analgesia depending on pain score/severity

(14) **Give post-procedural advice**
This should include caring for the scar and worsening care advice regarding signs of infection or wound opening

Source: All photos are original photos taken by the Author; Francina Hyatt

Source: Dougherty and Lister (2015); Fineout-Overholt et al. (2005); Fraise and Bradley (2009); Loveday et al. (2014); NMC (2018); Pasquier (2015); Preston (2005); Pudner (2005); Pullen (2003)

References

Department of Health (2011) *Application Package: Surgical Instrument Traceability Version 6*. Available at: www.gs1uk.org/~/media/healthcare-user-group/gs1_uk_hug_technologies_surgical_instruments_trace_doc.pdf?la=en (accessed 26 July 2018).

Dougherty, L. and Lister, S.E. (eds) (2015) *The Royal Marsden Manual of Clinical Nursing Procedures*: 9th edn. Chichester: Wiley-Blackwell.

Fineout-Overholt, E., Melnyk, B.M. and Schultz, A. (2005) `Transforming health care from the inside out: advancing evidence-based practice in the 21st century', *Journal of Professional Nursing, 21*(6): 335-44.

Fraise, A.P. and Bradley, T. (2009) *Ayliffe's Control of Healthcare Associated Infections: A Practical Handbook*, 5th edn. London: Hodder Arnold.

Loveday, H.P., Wilson, J.A., Pratt, R.J., Golsorkhi, M., Tingle, A., Bak, A. et al. (2014) 'Epic3: National evidence-based guidelines for preventing healthcare-associated infections in NHS hospitals in England', *Journal of Hospital Infection*, *86*(S1): S1-S70.

McClelland, H. and Nellis, G. (1997) `Surgical staple trial in accident and emergency', *Accident and Emergency Nursing*, *5*(2): 62-4.

Nursing and Midwifery Council (NMC) (2018) The Code: Professional Standards of Practice and Behaviour for Nurses, Midwives and Nursing Associates. London: NMC. Available at: www.nmc.org.uk/globalassets/sitedocuments/nmc-publications/nmc-code.pdf (accessed 31 October 2018).

Perry, A. and Potter, P. (2015) *Clinical Nursing Skills and Techniques*, 8th edn. St Louis: Elsevier Mosby.

Preston, R.M. (2005) 'Aseptic technique: evidence-based approach for patient safety', *British Journal of Nursing*, *14*(10): 540-2, 544-6. Available at: www.magonlinelibrary.com/doi/pdf/10.12968/bjon.2005.14.10.18102 (accessed 27 July 2018).

Pudner, R. (2005) 'Wound healing in the surgical patient', in *Nursing the Surgical Patient*, 2nd edn. Edinburgh: Elsevier, pp. 45-69.

Pullen, L.R. (2003) 'Removing sutures and staples', *Nursing*, *33*(10): 18. Available at: https://insights.ovid.com/pubmed?pmid=14571877 (accessed 26 July 2018).

URINARY CATHETERISATION
FIONA LUNDIE AND DEBBIE MCCRAW

☑ Before you start

Before you undertake this procedure a full patient assessment is necessary and consideration as to whether the procedure is required. Most placement areas/health boards/trusts require that qualified nurses undertake further training before undertaking this procedure.

☑ Essential equipment

Please review local policy and use:

- suitable catheter
- sterile field
- suitable personal protective equipment (PPE), in this case gloves and apron
- sterile gloves
- anaesthetic lubricant
- sterile water
- antiseptic hand gel.

☑ Care-setting considerations

In community settings a trolley is unlikely to be available. A suitable hard surface should be used although the cleaning of this with alcohol is unlikely to occur.

☑ What to watch out for and action to take

- The environment: consider - adequate lighting, ventilation, privacy.
- Positioning: consider - operator and patient.

- Anaesthetic lubricant should be applied.
- Check all packaging before opening: expiry date, packaging undamaged.
- Follow Moving and Handling policy.
- Ensure the catheter is fully in the bladder. Advance a few centimetres until urine drains freely via the catheter to ensure the balloon is fully in the bladder as trauma and pain can occur if the balloon is in the urethra when expanded.

☑ **Helpful hints**

- Gloves and aprons must be worn. Hand hygiene must be performed before touching a patient, before clean/aseptic procedures, after body fluid exposure/risk, after touching a patient and after touching a patient's surroundings.
- Waste should be disposed of in a clinical waste bag.
- Keep the catheter in the sterile inner covering and use this to prevent touching the catheter during insertion.

Male catheterisation: step by step

 The first step of any procedure is to introduce yourself to the patient, explain the procedure and gain their consent
Fully informed consent may not always be possible if the patient is a child, has mental health problems or has learning disabilities. Even in these circumstances, however, every effort should be made to explain the procedure in terms that the patient can understand. In the case of patients who are unable to provide consent because they are unconscious, advice should be sought from your practice educator or another registered nurse

 Gather the equipment required
Ensures you are fully prepared; also avoids you having to leave the patient or interrupt the procedure

 Clear sufficient space within the environment
This enables clear access to the patient and the nurse to safely use the equipment required

4
Wash your hands with soap and water before you undertake the procedure and ensure that antiseptic gel is available for use as required during the procedure
An apron should also be worn. This reduces the risk of infection

5
Draw the curtains for privacy or undertake procedure in a separate room
Maintains patient privacy, dignity and comfort

6
Ensure the patient is in a comfortable supine position and appropriately covered with sheets/blankets
Promotes patient comfort and reduces anxiety. Maintains patient privacy, dignity and comfort

7
Put on disposable apron and prepare trolley
This reduces the risk of infection and provides a suitable working area

8
If using a catheterisation pack, open sterile items and create your 'sterile field' by placing only sterile items within this area
Creating a sterile field avoids contamination through direct contact with non-sterile items. Remember, your hands are not sterile!

9
Undertake procedure, ensuring that only sterile items come into contact with the susceptible site and that sterile and non-sterile items do not come into contact with each other
To prevent and control infection

10
Open all other packs required and place on the open catheter pack, using an aseptic technique, leaving the urinary catheter in the inner sterile wrapping
Reduces the risk of infection

11
Using a sterile swab, grasp the penis and retract the foreskin if necessary. Cleanse the glans penis with sterile water or 0.9% sodium chloride
To reduce the risk of introducing infection

12
When catheterising a male, insert the tip of the syringe of anaesthetic lubricating gel into the urethra and slowly squeeze the gel into the urethra, keeping the

penis upright. Massage the gel along the shaft of the penis to ensure it distributes along the urethra
Lubrication prevents trauma and anaesthesia reduces discomfort. The penis will have to be held in this position for 3-5 minutes to ensure adequate anaesthesia. Prevent the anaesthetic gel leaking out by keeping the penis upright

(13) Remove gloves, cleanse hands with gel and put on a second pair of sterile gloves
Reduces the risk of infection

(14) Grasp the penis, raising and extending it
Straightens the urethra and facilitates ease of catheterisation

(15) Insert the MALE LENGTH catheter for approximately 15-25 cm until a flow of urine occurs
This ensures the catheter is fully in the bladder

(16) Straighten penis horizontally
To assist with insertion

(17) Apply only gentle pressure to the catheter if resistance is felt. Patient can be asked to cough or apply pressure (as if passing urine)
Helps relax external sphincter

(18) Once urine flow noted, advance the catheter gently and inflate the balloon as per manufacture's guidelines
Prevents balloon being inflated in the urethra, which will cause pain and trauma to the patient

(19) Withdraw catheter slightly until resistance felt and attach to urinary drainage system. Ensure catheter and drainage tubing and bag are fully supported
Ensure patient comfort, reduces risk of urethral trauma and encourages better flow of urine

(20) Reposition foreskin after checking glans penis is clean and dry
To prevent paraphimosis

(21) Leave the patient and immediate surrounding area clean and dry
Enhance patient comfort and reduce risk of infection and skin irritation

(22) **Ensure the patient is in a comfortable position, with drinks and call bells available (if in a hospital setting)**
Promotes patient comfort and ensures they are well hydrated

(23) **Dispose of all equipment appropriately**
To reduce the risk of cross infection

(24) **Record in patient documentation**
Type, size and manufacturer of catheter, plus batch number; reason for catheterisation and any problems encountered; type of lubricant used and batch number; date for review and future change date if required; amount of water inserted in balloon. To maintain patient safety and continuity of care

Female Catheterisation: Step by step

Follow steps 1 to 5 as above then:

(6) **Help the patient into a supine position with her legs bent and her knees apart (Note: If this is uncomfortable for the patient, help her to bend one knee and keep the other straight or to open her legs as far as possible)**
To ensure the patient is in the most suitable position for insertion of the catheter

Follow steps 7 to 10 as above then:

(11) **Using your non-dominant hand, separate the labia minora and labia majora to visualise the urethral meatus**
To allow you to view the urethra for catheter insertion

(12) **Keep the labia open with your non-dominant hand and, using your dominant hand, clean the urethral meatus using 0.9% sterile sodium chloride. Use only single, downward strokes towards the anus**
To prevent cross infection

13 Insert the nozzle of the lubricating/anaesthetic gel into the urethra. Leave for approximately 3-5 minutes to take effect (Note: You are able to continue with the procedure immediately if you are using only lubricating gel without the anaesthetic - refer to local policy)
Lubrication prevents trauma and anaesthesia reduces discomfort

14 Remove gloves, wash hands and put on another pair of sterile gloves
Reduces the risk of infection

15 Open the catheter, exposing only the tip and leaving the remainder in the sterile package. Place between the patient's thighs
To assist with insertion and to reduce the risk of infection

16 Hold the labia open with your non-dominant hand and introduce the tip of the catheter into the urethral orifice. In consideration of the female anatomy, use an upward and backward direction of introduction. The catheter should be inserted to approximately 5-6 cm
To allow ease of insertion

17 Once urine flow noted, advance the catheter gently and inflate the balloon as per manufacture's guidelines
Prevents balloon being inflated in the urethra, which will cause pain and trauma to patient

18 Withdraw catheter slightly until resistance felt and attach to urinary drainage system. Ensure catheter and drainage tubing and bag are fully supported
Ensures patient comfort, reduces risk of urethral trauma and encourages better flow of urine

19 Dispose of all equipment appropriately
To reduce the risk of cross infection

20 Leave the patient and immediate surrounding area clean and dry
Enhance patient comfort and reduce infection and skin irritation

21 Ensure the patient is in a comfortable position, with drinks and call bells available (if in a hospital setting)

Promotes patient comfort and ensures they are well hydrated

Document the procedure
Type, size and manufacturer of catheter, plus batch number; reason for catheterisation and any problems encountered; type of lubricant used and batch number; date for review and future change date if required; amount of water inserted in balloon. To maintain patient safety and continuity of care

Source: Delves-Yates (2018); Dougherty and Lister (2015); RCN (2012); Tortora and Derrickson (2011); Yates (2015)

References

Delves-Yates, C. (2018) *Essential Clinical Skills for Nurses*, 2nd edn. London: Sage.

Dougherty, L. and Lister, S.E. (eds) (2015) *The Royal Marsden Manual of Clinical Nursing Procedures*, 9th edn. Chichester: Wiley-Blackwell.

Royal College of Nursing (RCN) (2012) *Catheter Care: RCN Guidance for Nurses*. London: RCN Publishing.

Tortora, G.J. and Derrickson, B.H. (2011) *Principles of Anatomy and Physiology*, 13th edn. Hoboken, NY: John Wiley and Sons.

Yates, A. (2015) 'Selecting gel types for urinary catheter insertion', *Nursing Times*, 111(26): 18-20.

URINALYSIS INTERPRETATION

FIONA LUNDIE AND DEBBIE MCCRAW

☑ Before you start

Urinalysis involves recording of volume and physical examination of the chemical and microscopic properties of urine. It can go some way to assess disease, condition or infection and can contribute to the assessment of treatment given. It can also confirm or eliminate specific site as a focus of infection.

Urine voided first thing in the morning is considered the best sample to test as it provides the most reliable results.

Types of urine testing

- Urinalysis
- Early morning urine (EMU)
- 24-hour urine collection
- Midstream specimen of urine (MSSU)
- Catheter specimen of urine (CSU)

☑ Essential equipment

- Non-sterile disposable gloves
- Apron
- Urine dipsticks
- Appropriate urine specimen pot

1 **The first step of any procedure is to introduce yourself to the patient, explain the procedure and gain their consent**
Fully informed consent may not always be possible if the patient is a child, has mental health problems or has learning disabilities; even in these circumstances, however, every effort should be made to explain the procedure in terms that the patient can understand. In the case of patients who are unable to provide consent because they are unconscious, advice should be sought from your practice educator or another registered nurse

2 **Gather the equipment required**
Ensures you are fully prepared; also avoids you having to leave the patient or interrupt the procedure

3 **Clear sufficient space within the environment, for example around the bed space or chair**
Enables clear access for the patient and the nurse to safely use the equipment required

4 **Wash your hands with soap and water before you undertake clinical measurements**
Consider the individual patient situation and the risk presented

5 **Ask the patient if they wish to have the curtains drawn for privacy or, if not possible, to be in a separate room if required**
Maintains patient privacy, dignity and comfort

6 **Obtain a clean specimen of urine, which should be tested immediately or, if not possible, within 2 hours to provide reliable results as stored urine will deteriorate rapidly**
To ensure an accurate result is recorded

7 **Ensure the dipsticks are in date and have been stored correctly as per manufacturers recommendations**
To ensure an accurate result

8 **Immerse the reagent strip into the urine for 1 second then remove. Run the strip along the edge of the container**
To remove excess urine and to prevent the mix of chemicals from adjacent reagent areas

(9) Hold the stick horizontally
Avoid holding upright as this may cause urine to run between reagent squares

(10) Wait the stated time before comparing the strip against the colour chart. This is usually 60 seconds
Observe manufacturer's guidance. Accurate timing and recording of readings is essential to avoid inaccurate results

(11) Dispose of urine sample and urinalysis stick appropriately. Remove gloves and apron and replace sealed reagent strips as per storage guidelines
To adhere to storage guidelines and maintain infection control

(12) Wash and dry hands
To prevent cross infection

(13) Document urinalysis readings. Inform medical or senior staff of any abnormal readings
This will allow quick action if treatment is required.

Interpreting the results

(1) Colour: Urine colour varies based on the urine concentration and can contrast from pale light yellow to dark amber. Some medications and foods can affect the colour of urine. Normal urine is often described as straw coloured.

(2) Clarity: Sometimes known as turbidity. Refers to how clear the urine is. Can be classified as clear, mildly cloudy, cloudy or turbid.

(3) Leukocytes: Not normally present in urine and can indicate urinary tract infections, sexually transmitted infections or contamination of sample from vaginal secretions.

(4) Nitrites: Not normally present in urine and can indicate bacterial infection.

(5) Urobilinogen: Normal for urine to contain urobilinogen but not bilirubin (see below).

6 **Protein:** Not normally present in urine. Can indicate damage or disease to glomerular filtration barrier; hypertension; kidney damage or diabetes mellitus.

7 **Urinary pH:** Measures the hydrogen ion content of urine. Normal range is 4.5-8. Can be affected by diet and medication.

8 **Haemoglobin:** Not normally present in urine. Can indicate trauma, infection or contamination of sample from vaginal secretions.

9 **Specific gravity:** Measures urine concentration. Normal range is around 1.010 to 1.030.

10 **Ketones:** Produced during fat metabolism, and not normally present in urine. Presence in urine can indicate diabetes, alcoholism, eclampsia, starvation and pregnancy.

11 **Bilirubin:** Not normally present in urine and may indicate a breakdown of red blood cells, liver disease or bile duct problems.

12 **Glucose:** If present in urine, referred to as glycosuria. Most commonly noted as an indicator of diabetes mellitus but can be noted in pregnancy. Not normally present in urine.

Source: Dougherty and Lister (2015); Roche Diagnostics (2010); Yates (2016)

References

Dougherty, L. and Lister, S.E. (eds) (2015) *The Royal Marsden Manual of Clinical Nursing Procedures*, 9th edn. Chichester: Wiley-Blackwell.

Roche Diagnostics (2010) *Compendium of Urinalysis: Urine Test Strips and Microscopy*. Geneva: Roche Diagnostics.

Yates, A. (2016) 'Urinalysis: How to interpret results', *Nursing Times. 2*, 1-3. Available at: www.nursingtimes.net/clinical-archive/continence/urinalysis-how-to-interpret-results/7005353.article (accessed 17 December 2018).

SEPSIS

LIZANNE HAMILTON-SMITH AND MEGHAN BATESON

Introduction

Sepsis is common and deadly. It is defined as a 'life threatening condition that arises when the body's response to an infection injures its own tissues and organs' (Singer et al., 2016). It is a major cause of morbidity, mortality and hospital admission. Internationally early detection, management and escalation of people with sepsis can prevent progression to septic shock and save lives (Rhodes et al., 2017).

There are different approaches to the identification of sepsis and you should follow the local policy for sepsis recognition in partnership with your mentor. The approach discussed in this chapter identifies people suspected of having sepsis as those with a suspected/confirmed source of infection and a National Early Warning Score (NEWS or NEWS2) of greater than or equal to 5 (RCP, 2017). Please note that patients with a NEWS or NEWS2 of less than 5 may also develop sepsis.

There are several care bundles available to guide the treatment of sepsis. The one used in this chapter is the Sepsis Six (Daniels et al., 2011), commonly used in the United Kingdom. You must follow local policy and procedure for the treatment of sepsis in conjunction with your mentor.

☑ Essential equipment

Some clinical areas have sepsis trolleys that contain all the equipment required. If a sepsis trolley is available please use it as it will save time in collecting the required equipment.

- **Monitoring of vital signs:** Sphygmomanometer, pulse oximeter, thermometer, NEWS or NEWS2 chart or equivalent.
- **Oxygen administration:** Oxygen mask, tubing, oxygen point.
- **Intravenous cannulation:** See Peripheral IV Cannualtion chapter for cannulation equipment and procedure.
- **Blood culture collection:** Equipment for venepuncture (see Venepuncture chapter for detail), set of blood culture bottles (one aerobic, one anaerobic), request form.
- **Lactate collection:** Arterial requires equipment for arterial puncture plus an arterial blood gas syringe, venous requires equipment for venepuncture and appropriate blood bottle. Please check local procedures for sending to lab.
- **Antibiotic prescription and administration:** Complete and legible prescription, antibiotic, diluent, syringe x2, needle x2, fluid for IV flush, alcohol swab, sharps box.
- **IV fluids:** See the Peripheral IV Cannualtion chapter and the Intravenous Fluids chapter for step by step.
- **Monitoring urine output:** Intake/output (fluid balance) chart, urinary catheterisation may be required.

Sepsis: step by step

This step by step has been broken down into early recognition, early management and early escalation of sepsis. Prompt management of sepsis improves patient outcomes and NICE (2016) advocate treatment within 1 hour of identification of suspicion of sepsis.

All aspects of this process should be undertaken with the supervision and support of your clinical mentor/supervisor. You may not be able to actively participate in all aspects of this process as a student nurse but it is important you know about them.

Early recognition of sepsis

Does the person have a suspected or confirmed source of infection?
Sepsis can develop from any source: a common example is respiratory infection, e.g. pneumonia.
Be aware of hidden sources, e.g. community acquired pressure ulcers

If the source is suspected to be from an invasive device, e.g. urinary catheter, you should discuss potential removal and replacement promptly with your mentor and the medical team

Does the person have a NEWS (or NEWS2) of 5 or more?
The combination of a high early warning score plus a suspected or confirmed source of infection would raise suspicion that this person may have sepsis (NHS England, 2017)

Even if the patient does not have sepsis, a high NEWS plus source of infection indicates that they are unwell and require treatment

If the answers to questions 1 and 2 are Yes,
think sepsis!

Report to medical staff immediately using a standardised communication tool
Using a standardised communication tool such as SBAR, report your findings to trigger rapid assessment and treatment. Providing detailed information in a brief and structured way allows the person receiving it to prioritise their workload by understanding how sick the patient is

Example SBAR:

Situation: My name is (your name) and I'm calling from (insert name of clinical area). I am calling about (patient name). I am calling because I'm concerned this patient might have sepsis.

Background: Admission diagnosis, date of admission, relevant medical history.

Assessment: Most recent NEWS score. Potential or confirmed source of infection. Any investigations or treatment started so far, e.g. oxygen.

Recommendation: Please come to review this patient immediately.

Early management of sepsis

A bundle of care will commence immediately following positive screening for sepsis. The following bundle is the Sepsis Six (Daniels et al., 2011) with the additional step of obtaining IV access.

Administer oxygen as prescribed
Oxygen should be prescribed and administered to maintain SpO_2 levels which are normal for the patient (usually 94-98% or 88-92% for patients experiencing hypercapnic respiratory failure)

Obtain IV access
IV access is required for both obtaining blood for tests (blood cultures and lactate) and administering treatment (antibiotics and IV fluids)

At the time of cannulation, additional blood samples may be obtained for urea and electrolytes, full blood count and glucose

If you are not trained in venepuncture and cannulation, prepare the equipment for peripheral IV cannulation and request an appropriate person to cannulate immediately

Obtain blood cultures
Two bottles of blood (one for anaerobes and one for aerobes) are obtained aseptically. Ensure the blood cultures are then sent immediately to microbiology. The blood cultures will be processed in microbiology to encourage growth of any organisms which may be present in the blood. It can take several days to grow an organism but only around 10-15% of all blood cultures are positive

Also consider any other specimen cultures, for example:

- urine sample if suspected urinary tract infection
- wound swab if suspected wound infection
- sputum sample if suspected respiratory infection
- additional blood cultures from existing vascular access devices, e.g. central venous catheters.

Measure blood lactate
Lactate is a product of anaerobic respiration, that is, when cells are working without oxygen. A lactate of >2 mmol/L is considered elevated

Critical care area or emergency department: blood sample will be processed via an arterial blood gas machine

General ward: send as urgent to biochemistry in an appropriate blood bottle

Antibiotic prescription and administration
Antibiotics are key to management of sepsis by stopping the infection. Local protocol will be followed for the prescription and administration of empirical antibiotics

IV fluid administration
IV fluids will be prescribed and commenced without delay. Please refer to the Intravenous Fluids chapter for step by step

Monitor urine output
An intake output (fluid balance) chart will be commenced to monitor urine output

Urine output should be at least 0.5 ml/kg/h. If necessary, the patient may be catheterised to allow more accurate monitoring

Early escalation

Early escalation and treatment of patients who are deteriorating is linked to improved survival. Patients with suspected sepsis who do not respond to treatment within 1 hour or continue to deteriorate should be reviewed by a consultant. Critical care admission may be required.

Source: Daniels et al. (2011); NHS England (2017); NICE (2016); Rhodes et al. (2017); RCP (2017); Singer et al. (2016)

References

Daniels, R., Nutbeam, T., McNamara, G. and Galvin, C. (2011) 'The sepsis six and the severe sepsis resuscitation bundle: A prospective observational cohort study', *Emergency Medicine Journal*, *28*(6): 507-12

NHS England (2017) *Sepsis Guidance Implementation for Adults*. London: NHS England.

National Institute for Health and Care Excellence (NICE) (2016) *Sepsis: Recognition, Diagnosis and Early Management*. NICE Guideline 51. London: NICE.

Rhodes, A., Evans, L.E., Alhazzani, W., Levy, M.M., Antonelli, M., Ferrer, R. et al. (2017) 'Surviving sepsis campaign: International guidelines for management of sepsis and septic shock: 2016', *Intensive Care Medicine*, 43(3): 304-77.

Royal College of Physicians (RCP) (2017) *National Early Warning Score (NEWS) 2: Standardising the Assessment of Acute-Illness Severity in the NHS. Updated Report of a Working Party*. London: RCP.

Singer, M., Deutschman, C.S. and Seymour, C.W. (2016) 'The Third International Consensus definitions for sepsis and septic shock (Sepsis-3)', *Journal of the American Medical Association*, 315(8): 801-10.

APPENDIX 1

BLOOD COLLECTION NEEDLES

SHIELD COLOUR	GAUGE	LENGTH
	22G	1" or 1.5"
	21G	1" or 1.5"
	20G	1" or 1.5"

BD Vacutainer® needles are available with a 20, 21 or 22 gauge needle.

The higher the gauge, the narrower the diameter of the needle.

Colours are universal and can be applied to other vacutainer systems used in practice.

APPENDIX 2

FLUID STATUS ASSESSMENT

Patients requiring IV fluids should have a fluid or hydration assessment by senior medical or nursing staff at least once per 24 hours. Along with a physical examination, NICE (2013) recommends that their urea and electrolytes are checked daily.

Fluid status can be broadly categorised as euvolaemic (normal fluid status), hypovolaemic (dehydrated) and hypervolaemic (overloaded).

Euvolaemia: Patients with normal fluid status who are well hydrated and have no abnormal fluid losses.

Hypovolaemia: Also known as dehydration, hypovolaemic patients have too little circulating blood volume. The two broad causes of hypovolaemia are:

1 output too high: losing too much fluid, e.g. diarrhoea

2 input too low: inadequate fluid intake, e.g. swallowing difficulties.

Hypervolaemia: Commonly known as 'overload', patients experiencing hypervolaemia have too much fluid in their circulating volume. The two broad causes of hypervolaemia are:

1 output too low: unable to make enough urine, e.g. chronic kidney disease

2 input too high for body's ability to handle the fluid, e.g. advanced heart failure.

Indications for IV fluids

Drinking is usually the preferred route for fluid intake; however, sometimes fluids require to be administered intravenously. The three main reasons for IV fluid administration are:

1 routine maintenance

2 replacement of fluid loss

3 resuscitation.

Routine maintenance is for patients who are unable to meet their intake requirements orally. Adults require a routine fluid intake of 25-30 ml/kg/24 hours. Older or frail adults require less at 20-25 ml/kg/24 hours (NICE, 2013). Patients with hepatic, renal or cardiac impairment will have different requirements and should have their intake goals set and reviewed by senior medical staff.

Patients who are nil by mouth should be considered for routine maintenance if they are expected to be nil by mouth for longer than 8 hours.

Replacement fluids are given in addition to maintenance fluids to patients who have experienced either recent or ongoing fluid loss, e.g. high output stoma, vomiting and diarrhoea.

Resuscitation fluids are given in emergencies when rapid fluid administration is required to preserve the patient's circulatory system, e.g. major haemorrhage.

Fluid Types

There are two types of IV fluids: crystalloids and colloids. Crystalloids consist of small molecules, which means that the fluid can leak out of the blood vessels into the surrounding tissues. Colloids have larger molecules that cannot leave the blood vessels so easily, which theoretically means that a smaller volume of infusion is required compared to crystalloid.

There is a move away from sodium chloride 0.9% towards increased use of balanced crystalloids, e.g. Hartmann's solution. The contents of balanced crystalloids more closely resemble blood plasma than crystalloids such as sodium chloride 0.9% or glucose 5%.

APPENDIX 3

INTAKE/OUTPUT CHARTS

Traditionally known as fluid balance charts, the main purpose of these charts is the assessment of intake and output rather than just overall fluid balance. For example, a patient who has an intake of 400 ml and output of 400 ml in 24 hours has both an inadequate fluid intake and output but would have a neutral fluid balance.

 Identify people who would benefit from intake/output monitoring

Ensuring only patients who require intake/output monitoring have charts completed means that time is not wasted on unnecessary charting.

Patients who may need intake/output monitoring include the following:

- acutely ill or deteriorating:
    - sepsis
    - NEWS of greater than or equal to 5
    - up to 48 hours post-discharge from Critical Care

- at risk of dehydration:
    - temperature greater than or equal to 38°C
    - frequent vomiting/high nasogastric aspirate
    - diarrhoea
    - high output stoma

- o   large open wound/vacuum-assisted therapy
- o   urine output <0.5 ml/kg/hours
- o   requires assistance to eat or drink
- o   nil by mouth for more than 8 hours
- receiving intravenous or enteral fluids
- requiring a fluid restriction
- part of routine post-operative management
- urinary catheter in place (acute setting)
- acute kidney injury.

Please note this is not an exhaustive list and does not replace clinical judgement.

Document the reason for commencing an intake/output chart in the nursing notes.

 ## Setting a fluid intake goal

It is important to set a fluid intake goal so that the whole team, the patient and their families know what the aim is for the day and whether or not it is being achieved. Without a goal it can be difficult to realise promptly when a person doesn't have a sufficient intake.

- NICE (2013) recommends that a person should have a total intake of 25–30 ml/kg/24 hours in the absence of any significant comorbidities. This volume is reduced to 20–25 ml/kg/24 hours for older and frail people.
- People with comorbidities such as cardiac failure, renal failure, head injury, etc. are likely to have different fluid requirements which must be assessed and set by senior medical staff.
- Remember that included in the total intake along with any oral intake are drug infusions, enteral feeding and total parenteral nutrition.
- Some patients require a fluid restriction due to comorbidities such as advanced heart failure or end stage kidney disease. As far as possible such restrictions should be managed in partnership with the patient and monitored throughout the day to ensure that their fluid restriction is well managed.

The intake goal should be agreed with medical staff.

Know what you are recording on the intake/output chart

- As a general rule only beverages and soup are counted as oral intake. Enteral feeding and all IV therapy must also be documented on the chart.
- Check local policy about what is included on the intake/output chart to ensure consistency.
- Remember to document the drinks when patients are taking their medications!
- IV fluids should be documented either hourly or retrospectively at the end of every bag as per local policy.
- For patients who are set a fluid restriction, fluid intake may be more carefully documented and include items such as ice cream, yoghurt and custard.
- Remember that if the patient isn't able to take large drinks but is wetting their mouth, this should be documented to ensure drinks continue to be offered and to highlight low intake rather than a potentially uncompleted chart.

Documenting output

- Urinary output should be at least 0.5 ml/kg/hour.
- Please adhere to local policy relating to measurement of urinary output for patients experiencing incontinence.
- Other losses must also be documented accurately as close to the time of measurement as possible. Such losses may include drain or stoma outputs, vomiting, diarrhoea and nasogastric aspirate.

Identifying patients at risk

- Intake/output charts must be totalled at least every 6 hours to allow continuous monitoring of fluid status and early detection of problems.

Totalling should take advantage of existing work patterns, e.g. before the ward doctor's handover to the out-of-hours team, or before the day shift handover to the night shift, to help ensure prompt identification and resolution of issues.

APPENDIX 4

ECG INTERPRETATION

Heart rate

To calculate the heart rate from a rhythm strip printed on ECG paper:

- Count *the large squares between the peak of one R wave and the peak of the next R wave and then divide 300 by the number* of large squares to calculate the heart rate in beats per minute.

Regularity of the heart rhythm

Is the rhythm on the ECG regular or irregular?

- Irregular rhythms can be either regularly irregular (a recurrent pattern of irregularity) or irregularly irregular (completely disorganised).
- You can measure regularity by measuring the number of squares between the peak of one R wave and the peak of the next R wave and then checking to see if this is the same between the other R waves on the rhythm strip.

P Waves

- The P wave represents the spread of the electrical impulse across the atria from the sinoatrial node to the atrioventricular node of the heart and results in atrial depolarisation. Atrial depolarisation triggers atrial contraction.

- There should be one P wave followed by a QRS complex.
- Note the duration, direction and shape of the P wave.

PR interval

- The width of the P wave to the start of the Q wave is the PR interval.
- Represents the time taken for electrical activity to move between the atria and ventricles.
- A prolonged PR interval may suggest atrioventricular delay.

QRS complex

The QRS complex reflects the spread of the electrical impulse from the atrioventricular node throughout the ventricles. Represents depolarisation of the ventricles which triggers ventricular contraction (ventricular systole).

- Changes in the duration, height or shape of the QRS complex reflect alterations to the pattern of electrical conduction through the ventricles.

ST segment

In a normal heart the ST segment is a flat line between the end of the QRS complex and the start of the T wave. During the ST segment both ventricles are depolarised.

- Abnormalities of the ST segment are common when the heart is hypoxic (lacking oxygen), e.g. myocardial infarction.

T wave

The T wave represents ventricular repolarisation which triggers ventricular diastole. In ventricular diastole the ventricles relax and begin to refill.

- Changes in the T wave may reflect a number of issues including electrolyte imbalances (e.g. hyperkalaemia) and ischaemia (lack of perfusion).

12 lead ECG interpretation

12 lead ECGs provide detailed information about the heart, grouped by anatomical location. Experienced practitioners can use the ECG to diagnose conditions such as ST elevation myocardial infarction. Interpretation is beyond the scope of this book.

Reference

NICE (2013) *Intravenous Fluid Therapy in Adults in Hospital* (CG174). Available at: www.nice.org.uk/Guidance/CG174 (accessed 17 December 2018).